Alcohol Policy and the Public Good

Alcohol Policy and the Public Good

_Griffith Edwards
Peter Anderson
Thomas F. Babor
Sally Casswell
Roberta Ferrence
Norman Giesbrecht
Christine Godfrey
Harold D. Holder
Paul Lemmens
Klaus Mäkelä
Lorraine T. Midanik
Thor Norström
Esa Österberg
Anders Romelsjö
Robin Room
Jussi Simpura
Ole-Jørgen Sk(

WORLD HEALTH ORGANIZATION

EUROPE

OXFORD   NEW YORK   TOKYO
OXFORD UNIVERSITY PRESS

Oxford University Press, Walton Street, Oxford OX2 6DP.

Oxford New York
Athens Auckland Bangkok Bombay
Calcutta Cape Town Dar es Salaam Delhi
Florence Hong Kong Istanbul Karachi
Kuala Lumpur Madras Madrid Melbourne
Mexico City Nairobi Paris Singapore
Taipei Tokyo Toronto
and associated companies in
Berlin Ibadan

Oxford is a trade mark of Oxford University Press

Published in the United States
by Oxford University Press Inc., New York

© Griffith Edwards and the authors listed on pp. xi–xii, 1994
First published 1994
Reprinted 1995 (twice)

A catalogue record for this book is available from the British Library

Library of Congress Cataloging in Publication Data
(Data available on request)

ISBN 0 19 262561 6 (Pbk)

Printed and bound in Great Britain by
Biddles Ltd, Guildford and King's Lynn

Foreword

J.E. Asvall, MD, Regional Director, World Health Organization, Regional Office for Europe, Copenhagen, Denmark

From the public health perspective, it is becoming increasingly clear that alcohol consumption plays a major role in morbidity and mortality on a world scale. For a long time, epidemiologists and public health experts underestimated the impact of alcohol on health. This was due to attention being focused on alcohol dependence or on alcoholism as a disease, which previously determined much of the thinking about alcohol-related harm. We now know only too well that alcohol dependence explains only one part of the harm occurring in individuals and societies as a result of alcohol consumption.

Against the background of the growing awareness of alcohol as an important factor in public health and, thus, in 'health for all' policies, countries and communities need to rethink their response to these problems. For instance, the health ministers of the European Member States of the World Health Organization decided unanimously at the forty-second session of the Regional Committee for Europe in 1992 to enhance action on alcohol both at national level and at European level. They endorsed the European Alcohol Action Plan as put forward by the Regional Office. Eight years earlier the same forum had already agreed on a firm agenda for public health in Europe. They had formulated 38 targets for Health for All, relevant for the region as a whole and for individual countries. One of these dealt explicitly with alcohol; Target 17 mentioned that a significant reduction in consumption was to be achieved.

Although there is agreement nowadays among experts and policy-makers alike over the general strategies to be followed to alleviate the negative consequences of alcohol drinking, many controversies and doubts still exist concerning the right balance to be struck between different strategies and the best ways and means to achieve improvements in public health. To what extent, for example, is it possible to advise the public about 'safe drinking limits' without creating a climate of heightened alcohol consumption, or of acceptability of higher drinking levels? And what about the even more fundamental question: is there really such a thing as a 'safe drinking level'? Or do the many exemptions that one has to attach to that concept pre-empt its value as a public health message? Another question is the extent to which public health measures in this domain that have proved successful in one particular culture can be transferred to other cultures, and one should constantly bear in mind the different situations in developed and developing countries.

Ideally, science should be able to provide at least some basis for the public debate and for the process of policy-making. In the recent past, considerable progress has been made in the science that deals with alcohol and health. However, much of this science is scattered and hidden in publications normally accessible only to those in the inner circle of alcohol studies, or 'alcohologists' as they are called in some countries. It was therefore a highly laudable initiative that a small group of experts, under the leadership of Professor Griffith Edwards, took on two years ago. They set out to scrutinize this science and to distil from it what is really relevant for the policy-making process. They devised the Alcohol and Public Policy Project, recruited a highly international team, consulted with experts throughout the world, and brought together, in the course of less than two years, the essential and accumulated knowledge available in the world today on how to deal with alcohol. This book is the result of their arduous work.

The exercise that the group performed followed the example on the same subject set twenty years earlier. At that time, Dr Kettil Bruun gathered around him the best analysts of alcohol policy and research and they produced a report which, like this one, was published in collaboration with the Regional Office and entitled *Alcohol control policies in public health perspective*. Few books have had so much influence on the thinking and actual policy-making in this area. Its great impact was due to the authority of the group, to the very thorough way in which they did their work, and to the practical form in which they packaged their conclusions. Looking at the quality and the amount of the work done for its successor, *Alcohol policy and the public good*, I would predict that this book will make a similar impact.

I am very grateful to all those who have contributed to this book. It not only provides a solid scientific basis for the European Alcohol Action Plan, as endorsed by the Regional Committee for Europe of the World Health Organization, but also provides an objective analysis on which to build relevant policies globally. It represents, in a comprehensive and readily accessible way, all the accumulated scientific knowledge on this subject and provides very practical guidance on complicated issues to all those who are involved, in one way or another, in the making of policies and practices related to the consumption of alcohol in our societies. Also, lastly, it represents an exemplary model of the way in which top quality expertise can be produced through teamwork, dedication, and sophistication.

Acknowledgements

The preparation of this book has depended on the immensely generous support of a large number of individuals.

Those whom we wish to thank are as follows. Cees Goos (Co-ordinator, Alcohol, Drugs, Tobacco Unit, WHO Regional Office for Europe, Copenhagen), was a member of the project's initial planning group and gave valuable input at many later points. Alan Maynard and Colin Drummond attended a plenary meeting of the project's working group, and provided helpful position papers. A large number of people assisted in furnishing statistical data, which have been used in this book, and these include: I.P. Anokhina (Russia), T. Dasananjali (Thailand), S. de Paula Ramos (Brazil), H. Emblad (WHO Geneva), Michael Farrell (UK), G. Gonzalez (Colombia), Marcus Grant, previously at WHO (Geneva), D. Hawks (Western Australia), Anthony Hurst (UK), M. Hussain Habil (Malaysia), Nicolai Ivanets (Russia), N. Jeanfrancois (France), U. John (Germany), Patrick Kenya (WHO Geneva), E.A. Koshkina (Russia), J. Lehto (WHO Europe), A. Mohit (Egypt), D.P. Rice (USA), D. Seijas (Chile), N. Shinfuku (Philippines), Eric Single (Canada), John Strang (UK), R. Velasco Fernández (Mexico), and J.A. Walburg (Netherlands). Anthony Hurst gave useful comments on draft material.

The Addiction Research Foundation (Toronto), Department of Health (London), Finnish Foundation for Alcohol Studies (Helsinki), National Institute for Drug and Alcohol Research (Oslo), Society for the Study of Addiction (London), and WHO (Europe) generously provided financial support. Invaluable support was also provided by all those institutions identified by the authors list which allowed their staff to give time to this project and which in most instances provided travel money. The full team or the editorial group held meetings at: WHO (Copenhagen); National Addiction Centre (London); National Institute for Drug and Alcohol Research (Oslo); Addiction Research Foundation (Toronto); and then again at the National Addiction Centre. We are grateful to those organizations for playing professional hosts and for much personal kindness.

Finally and in a category of her own, we would like to thank Mrs Patricia Davis, who has with unfailing efficiency and patience, provided the secretarial and administrative support which has held the project together.

Contents

A note on the genesis of this book

This book derives from the Alcohol and Public Policy Project (APPP), an independent group of 17 scientists from nine countries who have worked together in collegiate fashion over an intensive 2-year period. APPP's formal definition is as a project set up by a contract with the European Office of the World Health Organization. The text has evolved through position papers, many stages of drafting, full project group discussions, the interim work of a small editorial group, and a great deal of networking. This participatory exercise has resulted in a text which represents the consensus view of its authors, who have contributed as individual scientists rather than as representatives of any organization.

The authors and their affiliations

Griffith Edwards, D.M., Addiction Research Unit, National Addiction Centre, Institute of Psychiatry, University of London, UK

Peter Anderson, M.Sc., M.R.C.G.P., M.F.P.H.M., Consultant, Alcohol Action Plan, WHO Regional Office for Europe, Copenhagen, Denmark

Thomas F. Babor, Ph.D., M.P.H., Scientific Director, Alcohol Research Center, University of Connecticut, USA

Sally Casswell, Ph.D. Director, Alcohol and Public Health Research Unit, Runanga, Wananga, Hauora me te Paekaka, University of Auckland, New Zealand

Roberta Ferrence, Ph.D. Senior Scientist, Addiction Research Foundation, Ontario, Canada

Norman Giesbrecht, Ph.D., Senior Scientist, Addiction Research Foundation, Ontario, Canada.

Christine Godfrey, PhD., Senior Research Fellow, Centre for Health Economics, University of York, UK

Harold D. Holder, Ph.D., Director and Senior Scientist, Prevention Research Centre, Berkeley and Visiting Lecturer, School of Public Health, University of California, USA

Paul H.M.M. Lemmens, Ph.D., Research Fellow, University of Limburg, Maastricht, Netherlands (and recently Research Fellow at the Alcohol Research Group, Berkeley, California)

Klaus Mäkelä, Ph.D., Research Director, Finnish Foundation of Alcohol Studies, Helsinki, Finland

Lorraine T. Midanik, Ph.D., Associate Professor, University of California at Berkeley, California, and Affiliate Senior Scientist, Alcohol Research Group, California Pacific Medical Center Research Institute, USA

Thor Norström, Ph.D. Professor of Sociology, Stockholm University, Stockholm, Sweden

Esa Österberg, M.Sc. Researcher, Social Research Institute of Alcohol Studies, Helsinki, Finland

Anders Romelsjö, MD, Ph.D., Associate Professor, Department of Social Medicine, Karolinska Institute, Stockholm, Sweden

Robin Room, Ph.D. Vice President for Research and Development, Addiction Research Foundation, Ontario, Canada

Jussi Simpura, Ph.D. Director, Social Research Institute of Alcohol Studies, Helsinki, Finland

Ole-Jørgen Skog, Ph.D., Scientific Director, National Institute for Alcohol and Drug Research, Oslo, Norway

1

Drinking and drinking problems: empowering the policy response

1.1 Empowering the policy process

Alcohol inflicts a costly and unwelcome burden on the majority of societies, both in the developed and developing world. Across space and historical time and within the context of culturally determined value systems, administrative formulae, and belief as to the fundamental nature of the target issues, these problems have provoked an extraordinary diversity of policy responses. The catalogue includes such remedies as: total prohibition; state rationing and state monopolies; alcohol taxation; legislative controls directed at licensing of outlets, licensing hours, or definition of the legal drinking age. Other policies have involved mass media information campaigns or general or school-based education, aimed at change in attitudes, knowledge, and behaviour, or have sought to deal with the social conditions which encourage drinking – the temperance movement, for instance, or broad community interventions. Warning labels, and the control of advertising, have also been favoured. Some policies target drinking beliefs or behaviours generally, while others focus on specific situations (drink driving, server training or liability, workplace drinking programmes, for example), or specific target groups such as the young, or pregnant women. Early intervention in the primary care setting and also more specialist treatments contribute to prevention, or at least to amelioration of the worst consequences. The total list of potential policies is even more extensive, and their range and inventiveness is continually expanding.

If in some countries and historical epochs the public health response to alcohol problems has been crowded, energetic, diverse and even confused, and a leading political issue, in other places and at other times (and to this day), the response has sometimes been remarkable not for the jostling of competing activities, but for the virtual absence of any purposive public health measures at all. The ebb and flow of alcohol problems are in the latter circumstances regarded as inevitable, and as being as uncontrollable as the tide on the shore, or as only to be met by a token activity and some lamentation. Alcohol policies are in those kinds of setting a matter of concern perhaps to agriculture, trade, tourism, or the Ministry of Finance, rather than exciting the activity of health, welfare, education, employment, or road safety.

Diverse problems will require a diverse mix of remedies (Moore and Gerstein 1981; *Alcohol Health and Research World* 1993*a*), and what is apt or acceptable in one place or time may not be appropriate or feasible in another situation. There are economic, social, and cultural influences which bear on alcohol consumption and consequent problems, which will remain outside the control of government and cannot be engineered. The unbending assertion which this book will make is, however, that responsible administrations can and should do better than passively watch the flow of the tide. The level of alcohol problems which a society experiences is susceptible to amelioration by rational policy action – there is nothing inevitable about the level of alcohol-related distress. That assertion is amply supported by material to be presented later in this book.

In support of its core argument this text will explore, point by point, how an extensive and international base of research and policy experience can today inform decisions. By the end of this book the reader will have been acquainted with what is objectively known about which measures, in which circumstances, are likely to offer greater or lesser benefit to overall or specific policy goals targeted at reduction of the alcohol-related burden. This exposition will also have served a purpose if in passing it corrects misapprehensions which in the past have too often coloured policy thinking on alcohol. Those faulty assumptions have included, for instance, the belief that the population's general level and style of drinking have nothing to do with the prevalence and incidence of drinking problems; the assumption that heavy drinkers are a species apart from the generality of drinkers and will therefore be uninfluenced by ordinary constraints; the belief that drinking adversely affects only a tiny minority of the population; the too-exclusive focus on chronic illnesses which are caused by drinking, with accompanying neglect of the acute adverse consequences and alcohol-related accidents; and the comfortable delusion that our own favoured beverage is not really 'alcohol', but an essential article of food or an emblem of national virtue (beer or alternatively wine, are often thus viewed in certain countries).

The task for this introductory chapter is to offer an outline of the arguments and structure of the book. The text will at a later stage be exploring many different and complex issues, and it is essential that at this early point the fundamental coherence of the total endeavour is delineated. To that end we will first address the 'why now' or timeliness question. The nature and diversity of the problems which can result from alcohol use will then be described as a basic mapping of concerns. Some of the common and key perspectives within which the ensuing chapters will conduct their analysis will be outlined, and a signposting of the content of the individual chapters will be given.

1.2 The science and policy connection: why it is timely to review the evidence

One reason for formulating an updated statement on the intersections between science and alcohol policy, lies in the extensiveness and sophistication of the research output which has accumulated since the publication in 1975 of the report entitled *Alcohol Control Policies in Public Health Perspective* (Bruun *et al.* 1975), which presented an analysis of the evidence available at that time. Not only has research expanded on basic issues such as the form of individual- or population-level risk curves for consumption and problem relationships, the variations which occur in the distribution of consumption within the population consequent on changes in overall population level of drinking, and the econometrics of consumption, but so also has the body of applied research which examines the efficacy of different kinds of policy interventions. Hand in hand with that latter type of investigation and providing its substrate, has been the increasing range of national and local, general and more problem-specific preventive policies. The base of practical experience has thus greatly broadened.

It is also timely to take stock of the theoretical advances which are being made. Much of the more recent research output has been in terms of further establishing the necessary descriptive groundwork, but even at this level new statistical techniques (advances in time-series analysis, for instance), have given more powerful means for handling empirical data than were available 20 years ago. In some areas there are in addition the beginnings of theoretical developments which contribute to comprehension of the multiple and interactive determinants of drinking behaviour and its associated risks. An example is provided by work reviewed in Chapter 4, on the relationship between change in population consumption and the likely influence on levels of occurrence for different types of problem.

Another reason for believing that it is now appropriate to attempt the updating which this book will offer, is an awareness that certain large background changes are now afoot in the world which will make the institution of effective policies no less urgent, but in some ways more difficult. Here we refer, for instance, to the changes which have been taking place in eastern Europe as former socialist block countries move to free market economies, with the ensuing commercialization of the production and supply of alcohol: drinking did, of course, often give rise to extensive problems under the previous regimes (Simpura and Tigerstedt 1992). The removal of tariff barriers within the European Community and the extension of Community membership are similarly likely to weaken controls on the alcohol market in western Europe. In Scandinavia and North America, market control mechanisms such as alcohol monopolies have been abolished or relaxed. The developing world meanwhile continues to be exposed to enormous pressures from socio-cultural and market forces which are likely to exacerbate the level of alcohol-related problems (Maula *et al.* 1990). Trade agreements which are driven by commercial interests too often ignore health and social consequences.

A further and very positive reason for the timing of an exercise in review and synthesis is that there is today an expanded and more interested policy audience to receive, debate, and utilize the science. While there is still some denial and neglect of these issues, in many departments of national and local government and at the international level, there is greater sensitivity toward the need to design and review alcohol policies in the light of objective evidence (Mäkelä *et al.* 1981; Single *et al.* 1981; Klingemann *et al.* 1992). The role of WHO should be acknowledged not only in terms of recent contributions, but over a more protracted period in relation to analysis and communications on the nature of alcohol dependence and alcohol-related problems (Edwards *et al.* 1977); in development and dissemination of treatment methodologies (M. Grant and Hodgson 1991), in the conduct of international collaborative treatment research (Moser 1980; Babor and M. Grant 1992); and in support of policy formation and health advocacy (Bruun *et al.* 1975; Rootman and Moser 1984; Farrell 1985; Grant 1985; Moser 1985; Walsh and M. Grant 1985; Porter *et al.* 1986; World Health Organization 1993). The promulgation by WHO (Europe) of the European Action Plan on Alcohol is an important example of an attempt to establish a regional policy framework (World Health Organization 1992).

Finally, review might be seen as opportune not only because of the need to take stock of what new is known, but also because of the benefits which will derive from identifying gaps in knowledge. If further progress is to be made those gaps must be identified, and remedied by the next generation of research.

We referred above to the 1975 *Alcohol Control Policies* report (Bruun *et al.* 1975). That volume provides a starting point for this review, but the research and related policy experiences have progressed so considerably over the last 20 years that it would be inappropriate to construct the present book in terms of a second edition, or mere updating. Rather than being constrained by the previous framework, we have sought to build on the past, but have in large measure approached the task anew.

1.3 Scope of concern: the nature and diversity of alcohol-related problems

1.3.1 *The nature of causality*

The phrases 'alcohol problem' or 'alcohol-related problem', contain an assumption of causality. Within these superficially simple wordings there lurk, however, complexities. Causality in this field seldom or never has single or simple roots, and more often one is dealing with a causal nexus involving individual differences and social context; remote as well as immediate influences; and pattern, duration, and intensity of alcohol use rather than just the fact of its use. Furthermore, causality here is often conditional; a given level or pattern of drinking *may* lead to a problem, depending on who does the drinking, their accompanying diet, where the drinking is done, who reacts to the drinking in what manner, and so on. Causality here is not a matter of Newtonian physics, and uncertainty is part of every equation. For purposes of this exposition it will therefore be useful briefly to dissect the meaning of 'relatedness' within the phrase 'alcohol-related'.

1. *Caused acutely or chronically.* 'Acute' problems require the ingestion of a certain acute dose of alcohol and perhaps in particular context or circumstance, but do not require chronic ingestion. An example of an acute problem is a fracture sustained by falling over when drunk. Chronic problems on the other hand require a continued level of exposure. Hepatic cirrhosis is typical of a problem belonging to this latter category. It is also possible to conceive of what might be called 'acute or chronic problems'. A long-standing drinking problem leads, for instance, to cirrhosis, but at a certain point a massive bleed from the oesophagus supervenes: acute problems can have a chronic background.

2. *Caused by what drinking patterns?* While two individuals may consume an identical volume of alcohol over a week or a month or a year, the person who drinks in binges may be more likely to experience certain kinds of problem than the one who divides the same total intake into smaller but daily doses.

3. *Drunken comportment.* The way in which an individual behaves while intoxicated is likely to constitute a further important determinant of problems, particularly in the social domain (MacAndrew and Edgerton 1969; Mäkelä 1978).

4. *Caused to the drinker or to someone else.* Alcohol may, for instance, cause a driver to be intoxicated, but the drunk driver may then kill a pedestrian. There are many alcohol-related problems which are inflicted on passive recipients: the family, the employers, or society pay the costs. These consequences are often referred to as 'externalities'.

5. *Caused by social reactions.* Some alcohol-related problems (cancer of the oesophagus, for instance) do not require social reactions to supervene for their occurrence. Others such as loss of job, imprisonment,

the children being taken into care, or the marriage breaking down, are problems defined or influenced in their causation by informal or formal social responses.

6. *The alcohol or the beverage?* In most instances the causal agent for an alcohol-related problem is ethyl alcohol, whether contained in beer, wine, or spirits. There are, however, some instances in which beverage type appears to be associated with particular pathologies. Beer drinking may, for example, be related to cancer of the colon. Contaminants such as methyl alcohol can on occasion lead to serious complications or fatality.

1.3.2 *Types of alcohol-related problems*

With the need for awareness of the complexities which attach to 'relatedness' duly borne in mind, this section will sketch out the types of problem to which drinking can give rise. The aim is not to provide an encyclopaedic listing of every possible kind of large- or small-print entry, but to portray the scope of the book's concerns. To some extent it is possible to indicate the relative frequency of different types of problem occurrence, but such relativities will vary across time, between countries, or within different sectors of the community. Furthermore, any attempt to place very different problems within a fixed hierarchy of relative importance would be handicapped by the arbitrariness of the criteria employed and the weighting given to them. Those criteria might, for instance, include: pain and distress or impact on quality of life; acuteness or chronicity; years of life lost; harm to others; costs to health or social services, or wider aspects of economic cost.

For problems experienced by the individual drinker, it is convenient if somewhat artificial to order the presentation under separate headings relating to the physical, psychological, and social domains. This is the ordering which we will follow below with a further paragraph dealing with the problems which the drinker's behaviour can set for other people. Pointers as to the relative significance of different problems will be given in terms only of such qualifiers as 'commonly' or 'frequently'.

Turning then first to the physical heading and as a corrective to textbook listings which identify only the more classic alcohol-related physical pathologies, it is important to stress the extent and diversity of acute adverse consequences of drinking, such as trauma resulting from road traffic and other types of alcohol-related accidents, injuries from fights, acute medical complications (acute pancreatitis or alcoholic hepatitis, for instance), and so on (*Alcohol Health and Research World* 1993; Klingemann *et al.* 1993). Alcohol can also cause death by overdose

(Poikolainen 1977). Acute complications may in some countries or regions account for a major part of the total adverse physical consequences of alcohol consumption. With that point made, it is also undoubtedly true that drinking can cause damage to nearly every tissue and body system with consequent long-term disability or chronic disease, excess mortality, and expensive diversion of health care services (Lieber 1982). Damages of this kind include those which affect the nervous system and cause brain damage of various kinds and peripheral neuritis (Victor *et al.* 1989); high blood pressure, heart disease, and stroke (Saunders *et al.* 1981; Preedy and Richardson 1994); abdominal complications such as chronic pancreatitis (Benjamin *et al.* 1977; Sherman and Williams 1994); and cancers of the oropharynx, larynx, oesophagus, stomach, liver, rectum, and female breast (International Agency for Research on Cancer 1988). There has been a slow accumulation of evidence to show that alcohol problems can also present in many other types of guise: skin disease (Higgins *et al.* 1992), endocrine disorder (Marks 1981; Van Thiel and Gavaler 1990), blood disorders (Lieber 1982), muscle disease (Peters *et al.* 1985), bone disease (Spencer *et al.* 1986), and disorders of the immune system (Dunne 1989), are some of the additional presentations within a list which continues to expand.

As regards psychological consequences, alcohol acutely impairs many aspects of psychomotor and cognitive function. Impairment of emotional control can result in violence to others (Martin 1992). Alcohol is significantly implicated in intentional self-harm and completed suicide (Murphy and Wetzel 1990; Hawton *et al.* 1989). A not infrequent consequence of prolonged heavy drinking is short-term memory impairment or, less commonly, a more distinct picture of dementia (Lishman *et al.* 1987). Familiar to the hospital, but not so prevalent in population terms, are such syndromes as delirium tremens, alcoholic hallucinosis, and withdrawal fits (Isbell *et al.* 1955; Schuckit 1985). Dependence on alcohol is a leading psychobiological complication which can supervene with heavy alcohol use, and then perpetuate heavy drinking with further risk of many associated problems (Vaillant 1983).

The social problems which can result from drinking are again many. They include failure in work performance, absenteeism, dismissal, unemployment, and accidents in the workplace (Pratt and Tucker 1989; Stallones and Kraus 1993). Drinking can result in debt, housing problems, or at the extreme, destitution (Baumhol 1987; National Institute on Alcohol Abuse and Alcoholism 1989). The relationship between alcohol and crime is complex, and the causality question should here be handled with particular care, but alcohol is directly or indirectly implicated in various types of offending, including crimes of violence (Pernanen 1991) and, of course, drink–driving (see Chapter 7).

The problems which the drinker can inflict on other people commonly include direct impact on spouse and children in terms of psychological or physical trauma (Martin 1992), as well as educational, social, and financial handicap (Sher 1991). There can also frequently be an element of inconvenience, damage or cost inflicted on members of the general public – the victims of drink-driving or violent crime, for instance, or the workmate who is involved in an alcohol-related industrial accident. Finally, under this 'externalities' heading, one should note the enormous debit for society as a whole which accrues as a result of the welfare, health service, insurance, enforcement, and penal costs associated with drinking and the costs resulting from loss of production (Rice 1993). This issue is taken up again later in the chapter.

It is possible to react to the foregoing paragraphs at the level of detail, but one also does well to stand back and view the material more in the round. In a presentation which is constrained by the formalities of science it is not improper to remind ourselves that within the abstract listings lie degrees and varieties of ill-health, unhappiness, loss, pain, deprivation, denial of self, family disruption, wound to others, and destruction. Much of the suffering is amorphous and inchoate.

1.3.3 *Clustering of problems within the individual's immediate experience or through time*

Survey data reveal some individuals who report that they have experienced only a single and isolated problem with alcohol over the 12 months prior to interview, while others will state that over this time they encountered several or many such problems (Clark and Hilton 1991). Across the whole age spectrum survey findings indicate that a large part of population problem experience relates to single issues or occurrences, or to experience perhaps of two or three problems, rather than to large co-occurrences within the given period prevalence time frame. Not everyone who is experiencing a cluster of problems over one 12 month period will be doing so over the subsequent 12 months (Room 1977).

Surveys do, however, identify a small sector of respondents who have encountered multiple problems over the defined retrospective period. Wyllie and Casswell (1993) have, for instance, presented data from a 1988 New Zealand national drinking survey which identified a segment of young males who were heavy drinkers encountering multiple problems, and who were worried about their drinking.

There is a proportion of drinkers who continue over time to go on encountering multiple personal problems with drinking, while also perhaps inflicting multiple problems on other people (Robins and Regier 1991). It is likely that a significant proportion of such drinkers are suffering from alcohol dependence, and thus get caught up in rather intractable patterns of harmful alcohol use which will continue to generate problem after problem, year in and year out (Edwards 1989).

If problem clustering is a phenomenon which can be discerned in survey results, it is also one with which the welfare worker and the clinician are familiar. For the family which is struggling to cope with chronic alcohol dependence, the fact that problems do not come singly is manifest. Public policies must therefore address both the reality of single or infrequent and disparate problem happenings, and the fact of clustered or persistent problem occurrence.

1.4 Indicative findings on the prevalence and costs of alcohol-related problems: some international data

What we seek to establish in this section is a picture of the costliness, in a broad sense, of alcohol problems to societies. Recent reviews providing an international perspective on these issues include Giesbrecht *et al.* (1989), and Helzer and Canino (1992). There is though no relevant and comprehensive world data base on which to draw, and there is in particular a dearth of reliable information from developing countries, from eastern Europe, and from the republics of the former USSR. Comparison between countries is made difficult by variations in definition, sampling, and methods of data collection. There may at times and for various reasons be a bias toward underestimation. There is, however, also a danger of problem inflation. Survey definitions of 'alcoholism' have sometimes been worryingly imprecise, with consequent estimates for prevalences which are unconvincing. Costs can be exaggerated (Helen and Pittman 1993; US Secretary of Health and Human Services 1994). The causal contribution of alcohol to any given pathology or event is often difficult exactly to determine.

For these and other reasons, we caution against over-confident interpretation of any individual piece of the picture which is sketched out below. The figures quoted will often best be regarded as indicative rather than as firmly reliable. At the same time and whatever its incompleteness, the picture which emerges supports the contention that for many countries alcohol sets costly problems of large and diverse extent. A much better international data base is needed, but on the facts available it would be difficult to assert that the concerns of this book are trivial.

1.4.1 *Cirrhosis: different mortality rates in different countries*

Cirrhosis mortality is a proxy for heavy drinking (Smart and Mann 1992), but cannot safely be regarded as a surrogate for all types of alcohol

Alcohol Policy and the Public Good

Table 1.1. Europe: deaths from liver cirrhosis per 100 000 living with age standardization for European population, and ranking from highest to lowest incidence. Statistics supplied by WHO, Geneva

Country	Year of report	Total	Standardized mortality		
			Males	Females	M/F ratio
Hungary	1991	54.8	79.7	32.6	2.4
Romania	1991	38.1	47.5	28.8	1.6
Germany, former Democratic Republic	1991	33.7	47.9	19.4	2.5
Austria	1992	28.2	41.2	16.4	2.5
Portugal	1993	26.9	39.3	15.1	2.5
Italy	1990	26.8	31.7	18.0	1.8
Czechoslovakia	1991	25.1	38.1	13.4	2.8
Germany, Federal Republic	1991	22.2	30.4	14.6	2.1
Spain	1989	21.0	30.0	12.9	2.3
Luxembourg	1991	18.7	21.9	15.4	1.4
Former Yugoslavia	1990	18.4	27.7	10.2	2.7
France	1991	17.0	23.3	10.6	2.2
Bulgaria	1991	15.0	22.0	7.8	2.8
Poland	1991	13.9	19.1	9.2	2.1
Belgium	1987	11.9	14.4	9.5	1.5
Finland	1992	10.7	15.3	4.2	3.6
Switzerland	1991	9.5	12.9	6.1	2.1
Malta	1991	9.0	14.0	3.9	3.6
Greece	1990	8.9	12.1	5.8	2.1
Israel	1989	8.7	10.3	7.0	2.5
Sweden	1990	6.8	8.8	4.7	1.9
United Kingdom	1991	6.1	6.9	5.3	1.3
Netherlands	1991	5.1	6.3	3.9	1.6
Norway	1991	4.4	5.4	3.3	1.6
Ireland	1990	2.9	3.1	2.7	1.1

problem. Furthermore, it should be remembered that the proportion of the total cirrhosis deaths which are due to alcohol as opposed to some other cause, may vary from country to country. Cirrhosis mortality is, however, a statistic which is widely reported, and comparisons provide an indication of the degree of variation in level of alcohol-related harm between countries.

Table 1.2. The Americas and the Caribbean: deaths from cirrhosis per 100 000 living with age standardization for European population, and ranking from highest to lowest incidence. Statistics supplied by WHO, Geneva

Country	Year of report	Total	Standardized mortality		
			Males	Females	M/F ratio
Mexico	1990	48.6	72.5	21.8	3.3
Chile	1989	46.2	67.5	26.5	2.5
Puerto Rico	1990	29.7	47.2	13.5	4.0
Ecuador	1988	21.7	28.7	14.1	2.0
Costa Rica	1989	20.4	26.7	13.1	2.0
Venezuela	1989	19.4	28.6	9.6	3.0
Argentina	1989	13.3	20.1	6.4	3.1
Trinidad and Tobago	1989	13.2	19.6	6.7	2.9
Cuba	1990	12.4	13.3	11.3	1.2
Panama	1987	11.6	14.2	7.7	1.8
USA	1990	11.6	15.2	8.0	1.9
Uruguay	1990	11.5	17.5	6.8	2.6
Canada	1990	9.3	12.7	5.8	2.2

There are many countries where routine reporting of reliable mortality data in relation to cirrhosis or any other cause of death has not been achieved, and we have not been able to quote cirrhosis mortality statistics for the republics of the former USSR, most of Asia and the Pacific region, Africa, or from many countries in Latin America. The available data are presented in three separate tables, (Tables 1.1–1.3). In each instance and for sake of comparability, standardization is to a European population base. We will comment briefly on each of these tables separately.

Table 1.1 presents cirrhosis mortality data for 24 countries which fall within the European region of WHO. The possible influence of national variations in death certification procedures should be borne in mind. The total mortality rates vary from a high of 54.8 (Hungary), to a low of 2.9 (Ireland). Not only those two extreme points but the whole distribution speaks to the extraordinary degree of variation between countires. The ordering from high incidence to low incidence cannot be explained in terms of any one factor: beer as well as wine-drinking countries can score highly; the highest entries include countries from both east and west Europe; the two lowest incidence figures come respectively from a protestant country (Norway) and from a Catholic country (Ireland). The male/female ratios

Alcohol Policy and the Public Good

Table 1.3. Japan, Australia, and New Zealand: deaths from cirrhosis per 100 000 living with age standardization for European population, and ranking from highest to lowest incidence. Statistics supplied by WHO, Geneva

Country	Year of report	Total	Standardized mortality		
			Males	Females	M/F ratio
Japan	1991	13.4	17.7	9.1	1.9
Australia	1988	8.1	11.7	4.2	2.8
New Zealand	1989	3.7	5.2	2.4	2.2

vary from 3.6 (Finland and also Malta), to 1.1. (Ireland). A systematic and scientifically rigorous analysis of the, no doubt, multiple explanations which underly this diverse national mortality experience is not available, and we offer these data at face value.

The statistics for the Americas and Caribbean (Table 1.2) again show large national variations – data on many countries are missing, and standardization to a European population base may be less than satisfactory for some of the countries cited. Latin American countries in general report higher cirrhosis mortality rates than the USA or Canada, while the two Caribbean countries on which data are available and found in the lower part of the table (Trinidad and Tobago, and Cuba). The male/female ratio varies between 4.0 (Puerto Rico), and 1.2 (Cuba).

Finally in this series of tabulations, Table 1.3 presents mortality data on three further countries, Japan, Australia, and New Zealand, with again a spread of overall mortality figures and with sex ratios somewhere around the middle range.

What is to be made of this extensive but still incomplete array of national statistics on cirrhosis deaths? The strong overall message must be that with cirrhosis mortality taken as marker, different countries are encountering astonishingly different levels of adverse experience with alcohol. The difference between Hungary and Ireland is a matter of almost 20-fold variation, but one might conjecture that the average citizen in either country is equally unaware of these facts.

As for the male/female ratio, the wide national differences indicate that countries vary not only in overall drinking problem experience, but in the way problems are partitioned between sectors of the population. The observed variations in sex ratios hint strongly at the need to look for social, cultural, economic, and historical explanations, for the different mortality rates seen between men and women, rather than just at a biological vulnerability explanation. In sum, these tables between them powerfully suggest that, whatever the country, national experience with drinking problems is not a universal and inexorable fact. It is not 'a given'.

1.4.2 *The prevalence of drinking problems and alcohol dependence in general populations*

The fullest research on this topic comes from the USA. Recent comprehensive epidemiological studies from that country include the Epidemiological Catchment Area Study drawn from five selected geographical areas (Robins and Regier 1991). This study employed DSM-III diagnostic criteria (American Psychiatric Association 1980), and found a lifetime prevalence for 'alcohol abuse', 'alcohol dependence', or both, of 23.8% for men, 4.5% for women, and 13.8% overall, while for 1 year prevalence the respective figures were 11.9, 2.2, and 6.8%. In terms of the world league for alcohol problems, the USA can be regarded as a middle ranking country (see Table 1.2). The lifetime estimate from this study is of particular interest, dispelling as it does any idea that to encounter a major personal problem with alcohol is only a rare occurrence. Complementary data from the 1988 US National Health Interview Survey (B.F. Grant *et al.* 1992), where a large representative national sample population was asked questions bearing on 'alcohol dependence' and 'alcohol abuse', using DSM-III-R criteria (American Psychiatric Association 1987), showed for 1 year prevalence a 3-to-1 male to female ratio for dependence and abuse taken together (13.4–4.4%). Also of interest were the reported age gradients: for instance, for men the 1 year prevalences were for age 18–29 years, 23.5%; age 30–44, 14.3%; age 45–64, 7.2%; age 65+, 2.8%. The conclusion that such prevalences fall off with age finds general support in the wider American survey literature (Cahalan *et al.* 1969; Cahalan and Room 1974; Clark and Hilton 1991).

Turning from the American experience to that of a developing country, a national household survey conducted in Columbia which used answers to the CAGE questionnaire to define caseness reported an almost 20% point prevalence of 'alcoholism' among male respondents, and a 4% prevalence among women (Rodriguez *et al.* 1992).

Some recent survey data from New Zealand are given in Table 1.4 which reproduces results from a report by Wyllie and Casswell (1989). Prevalence for alcohol problems are given for men and women separately. What is to be deemed a 'serious' problem is, of course, a subjective decision, but among men at about the 10% incidence level one begins to see occurrences reported which certainly cannot be dismissed as trivial. With 9% of men reporting their having taken a morning drink and 5% having experienced morning shakes, one can begin also to form an idea on the

Table 1.4. Prevalence of drinking problems experienced over previous 12 months, subjects aged 14–65, New Zealand community sample

	Men 14–65 years (n = 799) %	Women 14–65 years (n = 881) %
Felt the effects of alcohol after drinking the night before	46	29
Felt the effects of alcohol while at work, study, or engaged in household duties	28	14
Awakened the next day not being able to remember some of the things you had done while drinking	22	10
Been ashamed of something you did while drinking	16	9
Been involved in a serious argument after you have been drinking	12	8
Sometimes got drunk when there was an important reason to stay sober	10	4
Felt you should cut down on your drinking or stop altogether but been unable to do so	9	6
Taken an alcoholic drink first thing when you got up in the morning	9	1
Found that you need more alcohol to get the same effect from it as before	8	2
Been away from work because of your drinking	5	1
Had your hands shake a lot in the morning after drinking	5	2
Got into a physical fight because of your drinking	5	1
Been involved in a motor vehicle crash when you have been drinking	4	1
Stayed intoxicated for several days at a time	3	1
Been told by a doctor or health worker that the amount you were drinking was having a bad effect on your health	3	1
Been told to leave a place because of your drinking	3	1
Been involved in an accident while at work, study, or doing household duties after you have been drinking	2	1

Source: Wyllie and Casswell (1989).

probable incidence of alcohol dependence among men in this population: with respectively 1% and 2% of the women answering affirmatively to those two questions, the gender differences are evident. This survey also showed that 32% of men and 6% of women (overall 18.9%) met lifetime criteria for alcohol abuse or dependence. Survey data of this kind, whatever the country, tend repeatedly to point up the range, diversity, and commonness of alcohol problem experience within populations.

1.4.3 *Mortality resulting from alcohol*

Deaths from 'alcoholism' or 'alcoholic psychosis', or resulting from such a frequently alcohol-related pathology as cirrhosis, are in sum likely to reflect only part of the true total of cases in which alcohol is implicated as contributory cause of death. In many cases of death by natural causes including, for instance, pancreatitis, stroke, and various cancers, alcohol may be an important contributory factor, and it may also often be so in relation to death by accident, suicide, or violence. Figure 1.1 is reproduced from a recent French government publication (Ministère des Affaires Sociales et de la Solidarité 1993), based on data derived from INSERM (1993), and although one should as ever be cautious about the

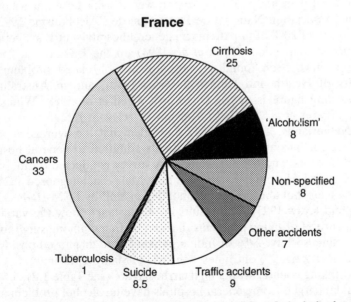

Fig. 1.1. Percentage contribution of different categories of alcohol-related death to the 70 000 annual total of such deaths. Source: INSERM (1993).

assumptions of causality which lie behind such official statistics, this pie chart indicates how different grouped causes of alcohol-related mortality may proportionately contribute to a national total.

1.4.4 Alcohol problems among psychiatric hospital patients

In Nairobi, Kenya, 21% of consecutive admissions to a psychiatric hospital were diagnosed as suffering from alcoholic psychosis (Badia 1985), while in Germany the percentage of such patients suffering from alcohol dependence has been put at 30% (Feuerelin 1989). In Sweden in 1983 (the last year for which data are available), 53% of men and 13% of women discharged from psychiatric hospitals had an alcohol diagnosis (Swedish Council for Alcohol and Other Drugs 1991), while for the Maudsley Hospital in London, the corresponding figure for in-patients and out-patients combined ran at about 10% (Glass and Jackson 1988).

1.4.5 Alcohol problems among general hospital patients

Turning from psychiatric to general hospital case loads, French data on this issue are revealing in that they illustrate the possibility of regional variation within one country. In the general medical service of a hospital in Toulouse, 25% of men and 6% of women were diagnosed as 'alcoholic', while 35% of men and 9.6% of women were so diagnosed at a hospital in Caen (Association National de Prevention de l'Alcoholisme 1992). In Germany about 20% of in-patients on general hospital wards are reported to be alcohol dependent (John et al. 1994), in the USA about 25% of in-patients have been found to have an alcohol-related problem (US Secretary of Health and Human Services 1990), and in Australia the corresponding figure is put as up to 30% (Bell et al. 1988; Williams et al. 1978; Ryder et al. 1988). In a review of relevant research conducted in the Netherlands, Zitman (1984) concluded that the average reported prevalence for 'alcohol abuse' for patients admitted to general hospitals was 20% for men and 6% for women. A survey conducted on the wards of the General Hospital, Kuala Lumpur, Malaysia, diagnosed 9.7% of patients as 'alcohol abusers' or 'alcohol dependent' by DSM-III-R criteria (Saroja and Kyaw 1993). The results in this instance show the variations in prevalence of drinking problems that can be found among subgroups in a multi-ethnic society: 22% of Indian patients were diagnosed positive on DSM-III-R criteria, 9% of Chinese, and 6% of Malays (Muslims). In Chile, a wine-drinking country with a high cirrhosis rate (see Table 1.2), 4.5% of patients discharged from general hospitals have an alcohol problem as the principal problem, while 38% have an alcohol involved associated diagnosis (de la Jara 1991).

1.4.6 *The involvement of alcohol in accidents other than road traffic accidents*

There are data available from several countries which suggest that various kinds of accidents can in sum make a significant contribution to alcohol-related morbidity and mortality. A recent Canadian report (CCSA/ARF 1993) suggests that alcohol is likely to have been implicated in 40% of deaths from accidental falls, 30% of deaths by fire, and 30% of deaths by accidental drowning. A summary tabulation of US sources gave corresponding figures of 28% for deaths by falling, 47% for fires, and 34% for deaths by drowning (Cherpitel 1992). Studies from various countries suggest that drinking is involved in 26–54% of home and leisure injuries (Honkanen 1993).

A review of research on the involvement of alcohol in emergency room attendance (Cherpitel 1993) which tabulated results from Australia, Finland, France, Mexico, Spain, UK, USA, and American forces in Germany, showed wide variations between sites. In nearly all instances where data were available, injured subjects had though a significantly higher prevalence of positive blood–alcohol concentration (BAC) readings than non-injured subjects attending the same centres over the same time. For instance, Cherpitel and Rosovsky (1990) surveyed eight emergency rooms in Mexico City, and found 11% of injured subjects with a BAC over 100 mg%, while only 2% of non-injured subjects gave a similar BAC reading ($P<0.05$).

1.4.7 *Road traffic accidents*

The contribution of drunk driving to the genesis of road traffic accidents is an issue which has attracted substantial attention internationally, and in many countries data are available on the BAC of drivers involved in fatal and non-fatal crashes. In Canada, among fatally injured drivers and for the year 1990, 9.8% had a positive BAC below 80 mg%, 9.1% a BAC of 81–150 mg%, and 27.3% a BAC greater than 150 mg% (CCSA/ARF 1993). In the USA in 1990, approximately 50% of such crashes are believed to involve alcohol (National Highway Traffic Safety Administration 1992). A national study conducted in France in 1984 showed that in approximately 40% of fatal accidents the person responsible for the occurrence had a blood–alcohol level greater than 80 mg%, whereas in Germany alcohol is believed to be involved in 19% of fatal road traffic accidents (Bühringer and Simon 1992). In the UK in 1990, 800 people died in traffic accidents where the driver was intoxicated, and a further 20 100 were injured in such accidents (UK Department of Transport 1991). Swedish data relate intoxication rates to the seriousness of the accident: in fatal accidents drinking is believed to be involved in between 7.1 and 11.5% of instances, but only in 6.2–8.7% of serious injuries and 3.7–5.6% of less serious personal injuries (Swedish Council for Information on Alcohol and Other Drugs 1991). There is little information on these issues from developing countries. In Chile, alcohol is said to be involved in 50% of traffic accidents (de la Jara 1991). Work from Papua New Guinea found that half of a sample of drivers killed in traffic accidents had a BAC of over 80 mg% (Sinha *et al*. 1981). These authors also reported that 90% of pedestrians killed had a BAC of over 80 mg%, with 55% at a level of over 150 mg%.

1.4.8 *The involvement of alcohol in suicide and homicide*

The findings bearing on these questions again require caution in their interpretation and the word 'involvement' hides real difficulties in causal interpretation. Recent reviews on alcohol and homicide (Pernanen 1991) show considerable variation across sample, country, and time. The Canadian estimate (CCSA/ARF 1993) that 30% of suicides and 60% of homicides are associated with drinking can be viewed as approximate, and is reasonably in accord with other research findings. Chilean data suggest the involvement of drinking in 38.6% of suicides and 48.6% of homicides (de la Jara 1991). In the USSR over 60% of homicides or violent assaults resulting in severe injury were committed by people who were intoxicated (Koshkina *et al*. 1994).

1.4.9 *Social costs of alcohol*

The overall costs to any country resulting from alcohol and embracing such sectors as health and welfare, loss to industry, costs from road traffic accidents, and enforcement and penal costs, set difficult problems, and published figures are best regarded with a large degree of caution (Harwood *et al*. 1984). Employment costs in particular seem dubious. Estimates have been offered from Brazil (Brazillian Association of Studies on Alcohol and Other Drugs 1990), the UK (Maynard *et al*. 1987), Australia (Collins and Lapsley 1992), Canada (Adrian 1988), and from Japan (Nakamura *et al*. 1993). The data given in these analyses are of interest, but given the qualifications that have to be put on certain elements which commonly go into their total, it does not seem appropriate to report these findings in full. Instead we reproduce as Table 1.5 data from a recent US estimate of annual costs under stated headings (Rice 1993): costs to industry were, in this instance, excluded. The total economic costs of 'alcohol abuse' to the USA for 1990 are estimated at over $100 000 million, with over 80% of these costs related to treatment, morbidity, and mortality. Whatever the

Table 1.5. USA estimated economic costs of alcohol problems 1990

Type of cost	Amount in millions	Per cent distribution
Total	104 918	100.0
Direct		
Speciality organizations	3 690	3.5
Short-stay hospitals	4 882	4.7
Office-based physicians	255	0.2
Other professional services	350	0.3
Nursing homes	1 165	1.1
Support costs	840	0.8
Indirect		
1. Morbidity:	38 965	37.1
Non-institutional population	38 728	36.9
Institutionalized population	237	0.2
2. Mortality	35 770	34.1
Other related costs	16 777	16.0
Direct		
Crime	6 178	5.9
Motor vehicle crashes	3 911	3.9
Fire destruction	673	0.6
Social welfare administration	128	0.1
Indirect		
Victims of crime	613	0.6
Incarceration	5 063	4.8
Special diseases		
Fetal alcohol syndrome	2 222	2.1

1990 costs are based on socioeconomic indexes applied to 1985 estimates adapted from D.P. Rice *et al*. (1990). Cost estimates recalculated from R.D. Rice (1993).

profits that accrue to societies from the use of alcohol, there are thus also likely to be substantial entries that have to be made on the debit side of the ledger. To try to balance the credit against the debit in terms only of economic calculation does not make sense – the cost to everyone concerned of, say, a man leaving a bar in a drunken state, and killing a pedestrian as against the tax taken from that man's drinking, or to give another example, the lifetime welfare maintenance for all the children who have incurred the fetal alcohol syndrome against the exchequer's profits from the liquor tax paid by drinking mothers. In social and human terms those calculations do not balance like against like. For purposes of the present exposition, the data given in Table 1.5 are entered simply to make the point that whatever the sum of suffering, alcohol problems also have a significant cost dimension that governments will do well to note.

1.5 Common and key perspectives

There are certain general assumptions which underlie much of the later sections of this book and it will at this point be useful to state them in outline form.

1.5.1 *Primary prevention of alcohol problems is a matter of salient public health importance within the totality of alcohol policies*

That goal will only be achieved through multiple rather than by any single strategy. This book will review a very broad range of research and experiences, but with a final common focus on how society is more effectively to prevent alcohol problems from happening.

1.5.2 *The word* alcoholism *is still widely used by clinicians, Alcoholics Anonymous, and the public at large.*

It has though no precise scientific meaning. For purposes of this book we prefer to employ the biaxial concepts of *alcohol-related problems* and *alcohol dependence* (Edwards *et al*. 1977). This formulation can help to bridge public health and clinical concerns.

1.5.3 *Alcohol causes problems but also gives benefit*

This book deals with the health and social problems which are caused by alcohol, and the policy responses to those concerns. That alcohol is also a source of enjoyment and a market commodity should be acknowledged, and health benefits will later be discussed in regard to the possible protective benefit of alcohol on coronary heart disease.

1.5.4 *Risk functions*

Today, this is a concept of importance to public health thinking (Rose 1992). Rather than a question being put in terms, say, of 'Does radiation cause leukaemia?', inquiry is turned toward what risk of leukaemia attaches to what level and duration of radiation exposure, and a curve describing the relevant *risk function* can be determined. In this book a risk function approach will be applied to the relationships between on the one hand,

quantity drunk, and on the other a range of physical and social consequences of drinking. We are not dealing here with inevitabilities, but with
assessment of the mounting *probabilities* of adverse outcome with graded
increase in consumption. As will be shown later, that kind of analysis can
provide information of considerable practical relevance to alcohol policy
formation.

1.5.5 *Continuities*

A continuity usually exists between moderate and excessive drinking, and
between harmless drinking and drinking which results in harm. Alcohol-
related problems present with a gradedness of intensity and clustering.
Alcohol dependence is distributed within a population in graded degree.
The individual furthermore often moves backwards and forward into and
out of problem experience. Thus what constitutes 'the problem' is a matter
of shifts, shadings, and degrees, rather than categories or absolutes or any
one fixed state called 'alcoholism'. If alcohol causes both pain and pleasure,
those two kinds of experience are thus not rigidly partitioned between two
different kinds of people, or two distinct populations.

1.5.6 *Policies will often impact to a greater or lesser degree on the totality of population drinking behaviours*

The impact may at one and the same time be on low/heavy consumption, non-problem/problem use, non-dependent/dependent drinkers,
rather than on only one narrow segment of any one spectrum.

1.5.7 *Alcohol dependence*

That alcohol is a drug which can produce a potentially devastating type of
drug dependence (*alcohol dependence*), is an issue on which policies must
take cognizance. In most parts of the world alcohol is a beverage constituent
which is licitly produced, supplied, and consumed, but the fact that it is a
drug of dependence (and one with toxic properties), must be taken into
account. Within that perspective alcohol is a rather special type of market
commodity.

1.5.8 *Treatment is important*

The alleviation of suffering through individually directed interventions is a
humane activity which not only meets individual and family needs, but

can have a public health impact by reducing the total sum of morbidity and mortality (see Chapter 9). The suitable population for prevention goes more broadly than the suitable case for treatment, but treatment and prevention are synergistic, interlocking responses to a spectrum of drinking behaviours and drinking problems.

1.5.9 *Small problems are important as well as big problems*

The population sum of lesser and preventable problems may in some circumstances exceed the sum of large and manifest problems which are of lower occurrence.

1.5.10 *Scientific findings bearing on alcohol issues may be generalizable between epochs and countries sharing common experience*

The likely generalizability will have to be judged in relation to a country's stage of development and other social and cultural factors. Generalizability will also depend on the particular type of finding. For instance, the relationship between drinking and violence may be much at the play of culture, while the risks for certain physical pathologies may be more culture free. We are particularly aware that nearly all the research and policy experiments discussed in this book derive from the developed world. Extrapolations from that base to countries where, for instance, a large proportion of the population's alcohol supply comes from home production or other informal sources is possible, but must be approached cautiously.

1.6 Signposting the chapters

The chapters which follow will be arranged thus. Part 1 presents a series of contributions which review important areas of epidemiological research. Within this section of the book, Chapter 2 analyses global trends in alcohol consumption and drinking patterns, and identifies some of the social and cultural factors which may bring about changes in drinking behaviour over time. Chapter 3 examines the individual's drinking and degree of risk, and this leads to a discussion in Chapter 4 of population drinking and the aggregate risk of alcohol problems.

With that basic groundwork established, Part 2 turns to research which has been applied to examining the efficacy of different kinds of strategy. Chapter 5 examines the effectiveness of taxation of beverage alcohol as an instrument used in the health interest. The impact of measures which have sought to control the individual's access to alcohol are reviewed in Chapter 6. Measures which have been directed at prevention of drinking in specific contexts (particularly drink-driving), are given focused attention in Chapter 7. Chapter 8 examines research on strategies which are directed at changing drinking behaviour through influence on relevant attitudes. Chapter 9 explores the role of treatment within the totality of public health responses to alcohol.

These reviews, both of more basic and applied research, lead up to Chapter 10, which in the light of those analyses will seek to determine how science can usefully contribute to the empowering of public policy. The aim will be to identify and assess multiple options, and develop a view on how strategies may be combined within a rational, flexible, and integrated policy response. Finally, in Appendix 1, thought will be given to future research needs, in terms not of an extended shopping list but of selected and major themes to which priority should now be accorded.

1.7 Whom is this book for?

A central purpose of this book is to inform and empower policy makers who hold direct responsibility for health and social decisions, to inform those who advise them, and to assist scientists who are engaged in researching these issues. Alcohol does, however, raise problems of pervasive significance for social action, social responsibility, social cost and public order, beyond the health and welfare departments, and affecting many different sectors including education and youth services, employment, trade and agriculture, tourism, penal services, highway safety, and departments of government concerned with trade and revenue. In addition, the ability of society as a whole, the media, and opinion formers, better to comprehend the issues which are involved is vital to many kinds of debate and decision. The book bears on these wide intersectoral concerns. We hope therefore that this text will be of interest not only to health specialists as narrowly defined, but to these many additional and highly important actors and audiences.

References

Adrian M. (1988) Social costs of alcohol. *Canadian Journal of Public Health* **79**, 316–322.

Alcohol Health and Research World (1993*a*) Prevention of alcohol-related problems. *Alcohol Health and Research World* **17**, 1–88.

Alcohol Health and Research World (1993*b*) Alcohol, aggression and injury. *Alcohol Health and Research World* **17**, 89–172.

American Psychiatric Association (1980) *Diagnostic and Statistical Manual of Mental Disorders*, 3rd edn. Washington DC: APA.

American Psychiatric Association (1987) *Diagnostic and Statistical Manual of Mental Disorders*, 3rd edn revised. Washington DC: APA.

Association National de Prevention de l'Alcoholisme (1992) *Document 35. 15 ANPA*. Paris: ANPA.

Babor T.F. and Grant M. (ed.) (1992) *Project on Identification and Management of Alcohol-related Problems: Report on Phase II*. Geneva: WHO.

Badia P (1985) Alcoholism among mental patients admitted to Mathari Hospital. Dissertation for Master of Medicine, University of Nairobi.

Baumhol J. (1987) *Research Agenda: the Homeless Population with Alcohol Problems*. Rockville, MD: NIAAA.

Bell J., The E., Patel A., Lewis J., and Batey R (1988) The detection of at-risk drinking in a teaching hospital. *Medical Journal of Australia* **149**, 351–355.

Benjamin I.S., Imrie C.W., and Blumgert L.H. (1977) Alcohol and the pancreas. In Edwards G. and Grant M. (ed.) *Alcoholism: New Knowledge and New Responses*, pp. 198–207 London: Croom Helm.

Brazilian Association of Studies on Alcohol and Other Drugs (1990) Project for a National Policy for the Prevention of the Consumption of Alcohol, Tobacco and other Psychoactive Substances. Document emanating from Agreement 11/90 with Ministry of Education. Brazil: Ministry of Education.

Bruun K., Edwards G., Lumio M., Mäkelä K., Pan L., Popham R.E., *et al.* (1975) *Alcohol Control Policies in Public Health Perspective*. Helsinki: Finnish Foundation for Alcohol Studies.

Bühringer G. and Simon R. (1992) Die gefahrlichtse psychoaktive substanz. *Psycho* **18**, 14–18.

Cahalan D. and Room R. (1974) *Problem Drinking among American Men*. New Brunswick, NJ: Rutgers Center of Alcohol Studies.

Cahalan D., Cisin I.H., and Crossley H. (1969) *American Drinking Practices: A National Study of Drinking Behaviour and Attitudes*. New Brunswick, NJ: Rutgers Center of Alcohol Studies.

CCSA/ARF (1993) *Canadian Profile*. Toronto: Canadian Centre for Substance Abuse.

Cherpitel C.J. (1992) The epidemiology of alcohol-related trauma. *Alcohol Health and Research World* **16**, 191–196.

Cherpitel C.J. (1993) Alcohol and injuries: a review of international emergency room studies. *Addiction* **88**, 923–937.

Cherpitel C.J. and Rosovsky H. (1990) Alcohol consumption and casualties: a comparison of emergency room populations in the United States and Mexico. *Journal of Studies on Alcohol* **51**, 319–428.

Clark W.B. and Hilton M.E. (1991) *Alcohol in America: Drinking Practices and Problems*. Albany, NY: State University of New York Press.

Collins D.J. and Lapsley H.M. (1992) Drug abuse economics: cost estimates and policy implications. *Drug and Alcohol Review* **11**, 379–384.

Jara de la J.J. (1991) *Los Problemas Derivados del Consumo de Alcohol: Medidas de Prevencion y Control.* Santiago: Documento Entregado, Por el Ministro de Salud. (Problems originated by alcohol consumption. Action on Prevention and Control. Santiago: Minister of Health document.)

Department of Transport (1991) *Road Accidents in Great Britain 1990. The Casualty Report.* London: HMSO.

Dunne F.J. (1989) Alcohol and the immune system. *British Medical Journal* **298**, 543–544.

Edwards G. (1989) As the years go rolling by. Drinking problems in the time dimension. *British Journal of Psychiatry* **154**, 18–26.

Edwards G., Gross M.M., Keller M., Moser J., and Room, R. (ed.) (1977) *Alcohol-related Disabilities.* WHO Offset Publication No. 32. Geneva: WHO.

Farrell S. (1985) *Review of National Policy Measures to Prevent Alcohol-related Problems.* Geneva: WHO.

Feuerlein W (1989) Zur Epidemiologie des Alkoholismus (The epidemiology of alcoholism). In: Schied H.W. Heimann H., and Mayer K. (ed.) *Der chronische Alkoholismus.* pp. 3–14. Stuttgart: Fisher.

Giesbrecht N., Gonzalez R., Grant M., Österberg E., Room R., Rootman I., and Towle L. (1989) *Drinking and Casualties. Accidents, Poisonings and Violence in an International Perspective.* London: Tavistock/Routledge.

Glass I.B. and Jackson P. (1988) Maudsley Hospital Survey. *British Journal of Addiction* **84**, 197–202.

Grant B.F., Harford T.C., Chou P., Pickering R., Dawson D.A., Stinson F.S., and Noble J. (1992) Prevalence of DSMIIIR alcohol abuse and dependence. *Alcohol Health and Research World* **15**, 91–96.

Grant M. (ed.) (1985) *Alcohol Policies.* WHO Regional Publications, European Series No. 18. Copenhagen: WHO.

Grant M. and Hodgson R. (ed.) (1991) *Responding to Drug and Alcohol Problems in the Community. A manual for primary health care workers with guidelines for trainers.* Geneva: WHO.

Harwood H.J., Napolitano D.M., Kristansen P., and Collins J.J. (1984) *Economic costs to Society of Alcohol and Drug Abuse and Mental Illness: 1980.* Research Triangle Park, NC: Research Triangle Institute.

Hawton K., Fagg J., and McKeown S.P. (1989) Alcoholism, alcohol, and attempted suicide. *Alcohol and Alcoholism* **24**, 3–9.

Helen D.M. and Pittman D.J. (1993) The external costs of alcohol abuse. *Journal of Studies on Alcohol* **54**, 302–307.

Helzer J.E. and Canino G.J. (ed.) (1992) *Alcoholism in North America, Europe and Asia.* New York: Oxford University Press.

Higgins E.M. du Vivier A.W.P., and Peters T.J. (1992) Alcohol and the skin. *Alcohol and Alcoholism* **27**, 595–602.

Honkanen R. (1993) Alcohol in home and leisure injuries. *Addiction* **88**, 939–944.

International Agency for Research on Cancer (1988) *Alcohol Drinking.* Lyon: IARC.

INSERM (1993) *Causes médicales de décès, année 1991* (Medical causes of death for the year 1991). Paris: Inserm.

Isbell H., Frasr H., Wikler A., Belleville R., and Eisenmann A. (1955) An experimental study of the etiology of 'rum fits' and delirium tremens. *Quarterly Journal of Studies on Alcohol* **16**, 1–33.

John U., Veltrup C., Driessen M. (1994) Alkoholabhaengige Patientinnen und Patienten in somatischen Abteilungen von Allgemeinkrankenhaeusern: Motivationsarbeit. In: Jagoda B., Kunze H. and Aktion Psychisch Kranke (ed.) *Gemeindepsychiatrische Suchtkrankenversorgung – Regionale Vernetzung medizinischer und psychosozialer Versorgungs-sstrukturen*, pp. 61–66. Koeln: Rheinland (Alcohol dependent patients in somatic departments of general hospitals: motivational work. Community. In Jagoda B., Kunze H. and Aktion Psychisch Kranke (ed.) *Community psychiatric Care for Addicts – Regional Network of Medical and Psychosocial Treatment Facilities* (in press).

Klingemann H.K.H., Holder H.D., and Gutzwiller F. (ed.) (1993) Alcohol-related accidents and injuries. *Addiction* (Special Issue) **88**, 861–1027.

Klingemann H.K.-H., Takala J-P., and Hunt J., (ed.) (1992) *Cure, Care or Control – Alcoholism Treatment in Sixteen Countries*. New York: State University of New York Press.

Koshkina E.A., Anokhina I.P., and Ivanets N.N. (1994) Problems of alcoholism and drug addiction in Russia. Working paper prepared for the Alcohol and Public Policy Project.

Lieber G.S. (ed.) (1982) *Medical Disorders of Alcoholism*. Philadelphia: W.B. Saunders.

Lishman W.A., Jacobson R.R., and Archer C. (1987) Brain damage in alcoholics: current concepts. *Acta Medica Scandinavica Supplementum* **717**, 5–17.

MacAndrew C. and Edgerton R. (1969) *Drunken Comportment: A Social Explanation*. Chicago: Aldine.

Mäkelä K. (1978) Levels of consumption and social consequences of drinking. In: Israel Y., Glaser F.B., Kalant H., Popham R.E., Schmidt W. and Smart R.G. (eds.) *Research Advances in Alcohol and Drug Problems*, Vol.4. pp. 303–348. New York: Plenum.

Mäkelä K., Room R., Single E., Sulkunen P., and Walsh B. (1981) *Alcohol, Society and the State 1. A Comparative Study of Alcohol Control*. Toronto: Addiction Research Foundation.

Marks V. (1981) Alcohol induced hypglycaemia. In: Marks V. and Rose F.C. (ed.) *Hypoglycaemia*, pp. 387–398. Oxford: Blackwell Scientific.

Martin S.F. (1992) The epidemiology of alcohol-related interpersonal violence. *Alcohol Health and Research World* **16**, 230–237.

Maula J., Lindblad M., and Tigerstedt C. (1990) *Alcohol in Developing Countries*. Proceedings from a meeting in Oslo, Norway, August 7–9 1988. English translated by L. Green-Rutanen. NAD Publication No. 18. Helsinki: Nordic Council for Alcohol and Drug Research (NAD).

Maynard A., Hardman G., and Whelan A. (1987) Measuring the social cost of alcohol misuse. *British Journal of Addiction* **82**, 701–706.

Ministère des Affaires Sociales et de la Solidarité (1993). *Alcohol et Santé*. Paris: Association Nationale de Prévention de l'alcoholisme.

Moore M. and Gerstein D. (ed.) (1981) *Alcohol and Public Policy: Beyond the Shadow of Prohibition*. Washington DC: National Academy Press.

Moser J. (1980) *Prevention of Alcohol-Related Problems*. Toronto: Alcoholism and Drug Addiction Research Foundation.

Moser J. (ed.) (1985) *Alcohol Policies in National Health and Development Planning*. WHO Offset Publication No. 89. Geneva: WHO.

Murphy G. and Wetzel R. (1990). The lifetime risk of suicide in alcoholism. Archives of General Psychiatry 47, 383–392.

Nakamura K., Tanaka A., and Takano T. (1993) The social cost of alcohol abuse in Japan. *Journal of Studies on Alcohol* **54**, 618–625.

National Institute on Alcohol Abuse and Alcoholism (1989) *Homelessness, Alcohol, and Other Drugs*. Rockville, MD: US Department of Health and Human Services.

National Highway Traffic Safety Administration (1992) *Driving under the Influence: A Report to Congress on Alcohol Limits*. Washington DC: National Highway Traffic Safety Administration.

Pernanen K. (1991) *Alcohol in Human Violence*. New York: Guilford.

Peters T.J., Martin F., and Ward K. (1985) Chronic alcohol skeletal myopathy – common and reversible. *Alcohol* **2**, 485–489.

Poikolainen K. (1977) *Alcohol Poisoning Mortality in Four Nordic Counctries. Alcohol Research in the Northern Countries*, Vol. 28. Helsinki: The Finnish Foundation for Alcohol Studies.

Porter L., Arif A., and Curran W.J. (1986) *The Law and the Treatment of Drug- and Alcohol-dependent Persons*. Geneva: WHO.

Pratt A.E. and Tucker M.M. (1989) Approaches to the alcohol problem in the workplace. *Alcohol and Alcoholism* **24**, 453–463.

Preedy V.R. and Richardson P.J. (1994) Ethanol induced cardiovascular disease. In Edwards G. and Peters T.J. (ed.) *Alcohol Misuse. British Medical Bulletin*, Vol. 50, pp. 152–63. London: Churchill Livingstone.

Rice R.D. (1993) The economic cost of alcohol abuse and alcohol dependence: 1990. *Alcohol Health and Research World* **17**, 10–18.

Rice D.P., Kelman S., Miller L.S., and Dunmeyer S. (1990) *The Economic Costs of Alcohol and Drug Misuse and Mental Illness 1985*. University of California: Institute of Health and Ageing.

Robins L.N. and Regier D.A. (1991) *Psychiatric Disorders in America*. New York: Free Press.

Rodriguez E., Duque L.F., and Rodriguez J.C. (1992) *National Study of Psychoactive Substance Consumption in Colombia*. Bogota: Fundación Santafé de Bogotá-Escuela Colombiana de Medicina.

Room R. (1977) Measurement and distribution of drinking patterns and problems in general populations. In Edwards G., Gross M.M., Keller M., Moser J., and Room R. (ed.) *Alcohol-Related Disabilities*, pp. 61–88. WHO Offset Publication No. 32. Geneva: WHO.

Rootman I. and Moser J. (1984) *Guidelines for Investigating Alcohol Problems and Developing Appropriate Responses*. Geneva: WHO.

Rose, G. (1992) *The Strategy of Preventive Medicine*. Oxford University Press.

Ryder D., Lenton S., Harrison S., and Dorricott J (1988) Alcohol-related problems in a general hospital and a general practice: screening and the preventive paradox. *Medical Journal of Australia* **149**, 350–360.

Saroja K.I. and Kyaw O. (1993) Pattern of alcoholism in the general hospital, Kuala Lumpur. *Medical Journal of Malaysia* **48**, 129–134.

Saunders J.B., Beevers D.G., and Paton A. (1981) Alcohol induced hypertension. *Lancet* **ii**, 653–656.

Schuckit M.A. (1985) *Drug and Alcohol Abuse: A Clinical Guide to Diagnosis and Treatment*, 2nd edn. New York: Plenum.

Secretary of State for Health and Human Services (1994) *Alcohol and Health: Eighth Special Report to Congress*. Rockville, MD: NIAAA.

Sher K.J. (1991) *Children of Alcoholics: a critical appraisal of theory and research*. University of Chicago Press.

Sherman D.I.N. and Williams R. (1994) Liver damage: mechanisms and management, in Edwards G. and and Peters T.J. (eds) *Alcohol Misuse. British Medical Bulletin 50*, pp. 124–38. London: Churchill Livingstone.

Sinha S.N., Seengupta S.K., and Purohit R.C. (1981) A five year review of deaths following trauma. Papua New Guinea. *Medical Journal* **24**, 222–228.

Simpura J. and Tigerstedt C. (ed.) (1992) *Social Problems around the Baltic Sea*. NAD Publication No. 21. Helsinki: Nordic Council for Alcohol and Drug Research.

Single E., Giesbrecht N., and Eakins B. (ed.) (1981) *Alcohol, Society and the State 2. A Social History of Control Policy in Seven Countries*. Toronto: Addiction Research Foundation.

Smart R.G. and Mann R.E. (1992) Alcohol and the epidemiology of liver cirrhosis. *Alcohol Health and Research World* **16**, 217–222.

Spencer H., Rubio E., Indreika M., and Seitman A. (1986) Chronic alcoholism, frequently overlooked cause of osteoporosis in men. *American Journal of Medicine* **80**, 393–397.

Stallones L. and Kraus J.F. (1993) The occurrence and epidemiologic features of alcohol-related occupational injuries. *Addiction* **88**, 945–951.

Swedish Council for Information on Alcohol and Other Drugs (1991) *Trends in Alcohol and Drug Use in Sweden*. Stockholm: Swedish Council.

US Secretary of Health and Human Services (1990) *Epidemiology in Alcohol and Health (Seventh Special Report to US Congress)*, pp. 13–68. Rockville, MD: US Department of Health and Human Services.

Vaillant G.E. (1983) *The Natural History of Alcoholism: Causes, Patterns, and Paths to Recovery*. Cambridge, MA: Harvard University Press.

Van Thiel, D.H. and Gavaler, J.S. (1990). Endocrine consequences of alcohol abuse. *Alcohol and Alcoholism*, **25**, 341–4.

Victor M., Adams R.D. and Collins G.H. (1989) *The Wernicke–Korsakoff Syndrome and Related Neurological Disorders due to Alcoholism and Malnutrition*, 2nd edn. Philadelphia: F.A. Davies.

Walsh B. and Grant M. (1985) *Public Health Implications of Alcohol Production and Trade*. WHO Offset Publication No. 88. Geneva: WHO.

Williams A.T., Burns F.H., and Morey S (1978) Prevalence of alcoholism in a Sydney teaching hospital: some aspects. *Medical Journal of Australia* **2**, 608–611.

World Health Organization (1992) *European Alcohol Action Plan*. Copenhagen: World Health Organization Regional Office for Europe. Document EUR/RC42/8.

World Health Organization (1993) *WHO Expert Committee on Drug Dependence: Twenty-eighth Report*. WHO Technical Report Series 836. Geneva: WHO.

Wyllie A. and Casswell S. (1989) *Drinking in New Zealand: A Survey 1988*. Auckland Alcohol Research Unit.

Wyllie A. and Casswell S. (1993) Identifying target segments of male drinkers for health promotion. *Health Promotion International* **8**, 249–261.

Zitman F.G. (1984) Het voorkomen van alcoholmisbruik bij in een ziekenhuis opgenomen patiënten. (The incidence of alcohol abuse among patients admitted to general hospitals). In: Geerlings P.J. *Herkenning en behandeling van alkoholmisbruik* (Prevention and treatment of alcohol problems) pp. 43–49. Universiteit van Leiden, Boerhaave Commissie. Faculteit Geneeskunde.

Part I

The individual's drinking, population consumption levels, and the risk relationships

2

International trends in alcohol consumption and drinking patterns

The brevity of this chapter has more to do with the paucity of the data base than the importance of the topic. Its focus is on international trends, and on the individual country as unit of analysis, in regard to change in per capita consumption and drinking patterns over time. Given that the expositions and arguments of Chapters 3 and 4 lead up to the conclusion that aggregate consumption and drinking patterns are likely to have a significant bearing on public health and welfare, levels of drinking and changes in alcohol consumption are matters of world-wide importance.

Levels and patterns of drinking are not set once and for all. In the first section of this chapter (2.1), long-term or historical fluctuations in per capita consumption are discussed. In Section 2.2, empirical evidence will be presented on more recent trends. Reliable data are available here mainly for European Community countries, but the information which is to hand on former socialist countries in Europe (Lehto and Moskalewicz 1994) and from the developing world will also be noted. Section 2.3 briefly discusses change in drinking patterns rather than overall consumption, while in 2.4 a note is given on change which may occur differentially with different population sectors within one country. With the factual basis thus outlined we will give a short overall summary on the types and diversity of change or stability which contribute to the current picture of the world's drinking, so far as it can be ascertained.

2.1 Historical fluctuations in drinking

Historical data vividly illustrate the possibility of large-scale ebb and flow in overall consumption over time together with shifts in beverage choice (Wilson 1940; Spring and Buss 1977; Negrete 1980; Room 1991). By the middle of the nineteenth century, alcohol intake was at a high level in most countries in Europe and North America. At the turn of that century, there was a general decline in consumption which continued until the period between the two world wars. The downward tendency was particularly marked for distilled beverages. It was also more pronounced in the spirit-drinking countries of northern and eastern Europe than in areas where wine was used on a daily basis. Nevertheless, a declining consumption was recorded roughly within the same time period in countries at different stages of economic development and representing a wide variety of alcohol cultures (Mäkelä *et al.* 1981). In France, which had reached an unprecedently high consumption at the end of the nineteenth century, consumption stayed at a high level (except during wartime privations) until the 1950s, since when consumption levels have shown a slow sustained fall.

Between the end of the Second World War and the 1970s, consumption increased in almost all countries which were able to offer reasonably accurate statistics, with some approaching the peak levels of the nineteenth century (Sulkunen 1976). In most countries, the rate of increase in consumption then slowed, while in some countries consumption levelled off or slightly declined.

Trends in consumption between 1945 and the early 1970s have been analysed by Sulkunen (1983). During this period, the largest growth rates were recorded in countries that started from a relatively low level, with the result that, in relative terms, the differences in average consumption between countries narrowed. There was also a tendency for countries to become more alike in their patterns of beverage choice, and the dominance of any beverage type relative to others often became less pronounced. Despite the trend toward convergence, there remained, however, some strong national differences in choice of beverage. The traditional beverages were not necessarily replaced by other drinks; the change was more one of addition rather than substitution. What is to be deemed 'traditional' within any country is a judgement which is likely to be in some degree time bound.

Such long-term fluctuations in alcohol consumption are notable in at least two respects. First, they are surprisingly common across countries, despite differences in economic development and the place of alcohol within the culture. Second, among the factors commonly put forward as explanations for drinking or problematic drinking (buying power, the amount of leisure time, social misery, or industrialization and urbanization, and so on), no single determinant shows consistent patterns of variation over time similar to the shifts in alcohol consumption. Levels of drinking are most often determined through the complex interplay of a wide range of factors.

2.2 Drinking trends in the 1970s and 1980s

2.2.1 *OECD countries*

Table 2.1 presents information on recorded alcohol consumption in 23 OECD countries in 1970, 1980, and 1990 (World Drink Trends 1992). The choice of these three time points is arbitrary, but changes over this

Table 2.1. *Per capita alcohol consumption (litres of ethanol) in OECD countries, 1970–1990*

	1970	1980	1990
Australia	8.1	9.6	8.4
Austria	10.5	11.0	10.4
Belgium	8.9	10.8	9.9
Canada	6.1	8.6	7.5
Denmark	6.8	9.1	9.9
Finland	4.4	6.4	7.7
France	16.2	14.9	12.7
Germany	10.3	11.4	10.6
Great Britain	5.3	7.3	7.6
Iceland	3.2	3.9	3.9
Ireland	5.9	7.3	7.2
Italy	13.7	13.0	8.7
Japan	4.6	5.4	6.5
Luxembourg	10.0	10.9	12.2
Netherlands	5.6	8.8	8.2
New Zealand	7.6	9.6	7.8
Norway	3.6	4.6	4.1
Portugal	9.9	11.0	9.8
Spain	11.6	13.6	10.8
Sweden	5.8	5.7	5.5
Switzerland	10.7	10.8	10.8
Turkey	0.5	0.7	0.6
United States of America	6.7	8.2	7.5

particular period are usefully illustrative of the kinds of consumption change which may generally be observed over the medium term. Over the two decades, France, Italy, and Sweden experienced a continuing decrease. In 15 countries, consumption continued to grow in the 1970s but decreased or remained stable in the 1980s. Only in Denmark, Finland, Great Britain, Japan, and Luxembourg did consumption continue to increase in the 1980s. The diversity of consumption trends in the 1980s does not rule out the possibility that in a longer historical perspective convergent trends might become evident. Indeed, one likely interpretation is that the post-war era of continuous consumption growth in the industrial world has reached its turning point, but with a slightly different timing in different countries.

As already mentioned, the post-war increase in alcohol consumption in the industrialized countries was accompanied by a cross-national convergence of aggregate consumption levels. This process continued in the 1970s

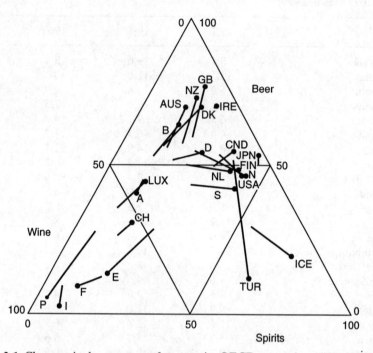

Fig. 2.1 Changes in beverage preferences in OECD countries 1970–1990. See text for full explanation. Each line shows for individual key country the vector of change, with · marking the start at 1970. Country symbols as follows: Australia (AUS), Austria (A), Belgium (B), Canada (CND), Denmark (DK), Finland (FIN), France (F), Germany (D), Great Britain (GB), Iceland (ICE), Ireland (IRE), Italy (I), Japan (JPN), Luxembourg (LUX), The Netherlands (NL), New Zealand (NZ), Norway (N), Portugal (P), Spain (E), Sweden (S), Switzerland (CH), Turkey (TUR), and, USA.

and 1980s. The countries experiencing the most marked decreases had started from a relatively high level of consumption, whereas the countries showing the biggest increases belonged to the low consumption countries in 1970. Cross-national differences thus have continued to diminish. The most recent changes in beverage preferences are shown in Fig. 2.1. In this diagram countries where the share of beer is more than 50% are located at the top corner of the triangle. Countries in which wine and spirits are the predominant beverages are in the lower left- and right-hand corners respectively. In the middle is an area where none of the beverages has a share of more than 50%. The starting point (1970) is in every instance denoted by the legend identifying the country, with the line denoting the vector for 1970–1990. The figure shows that homogenization has continued in the last two decades. With few exceptions, the lines depicting change move away from the corners where one beverage type dominates over the others. The general direction of the movements is not, however, towards the centre of the diagram (where the shares of all three beverage groups would be equal), but roughly towards the point corresponding to a beverage mix of 50% beer, 35% wine, and 15% distilled beverages.

In the recent period of more stabilized consumption, substitution has been more common than addition. In wine countries, the changes can be described as subtraction, as the decrease in wine consumption is only partly compensated by increase in beer and spirits drinking.

2.2.2 *Central and eastern European countries*

In many central and eastern European countries, social and economic upheavals threaten the reliability of alcohol statistics, and changing political borders hamper comparisons over time. In the former Soviet republics, recorded consumption fell sharply as a consequence of the 1985 anti-alcohol campaign. Despite widespread illicit alcohol production, the total decline in commercial beverage consumption was not compensated by increased home distillation. After 1987 and the discontinuation of the anti-alcohol policy, alcohol consumption again started to grow. Somewhat later, social and economic changes greatly increased the availability of alcohol in most of the former Soviet republics (Lehto and Moskalewicz 1994), but due to increasing private commercial initiatives the proportion of the total consumption covered by official figures may even be below that achieved in 1987. Rates for various indicators of drinking problems are, however, increasing in Russia, in the Ukraine, and in Estonia.

Since 1990, Polish alcohol statistics have covered only domestic beverages, while imported beverages remain unrecorded. Data from drinking surveys indicate a 50% increase in alcohol consumption between 1989 and 1992. This estimate is corroborated by a corresponding increase in hospitalizations for alcoholic psychosis. In the Czech Republic, in Slovakia, and in Bulgaria, alcohol consumption is similarly increasing (Lehto and Moskalewicz 1994).

2.2.3 *Developing countries*

Most developing countries are experiencing such intense demands as to make collection of routine statistics difficult or impossible. Reliable data on alcohol consumption are seldom available. A report by Walsh and Grant (1985) did not include data on non-commercial production, legal or illegal, but the authors concluded that 'the production and consumption of beer, wine and spirits are increasing in virtually all regions of the world', with the wine-drinking countries of France, Italy, Portugal, and certain North African states being the exception. There are also data to show that beer consumption increased markedly from 1960 to 1980 in many countries of Central and South America, Africa, and Asia. Corresponding information on wine and spirits is not available (Kortteinen 1988; Maula *et al.* 1990).

Smart (1991) reported that many developing countries showed large increases in commercially produced and distributed alcohol consumption from 1970 to 1980. However, the increase for African countries taken together was negligible, and there was only a slight rise in South Africa. Increases in Asia, North America, and Europe were substantial. Based on the information presently at hand, it is doubtful whether anything reliable can be said about drinking trends in the developing world.

2.3 Drinking patterns and changes of aggregate consumption

Changes in aggregate consumption may occur in several ways. New drinkers may be recruited from groups previously abstaining from alcohol, or a contrary process of abandoning drinking may take place as a consequence of increasing health consciousness. Drinking frequency and intake on an occasion may change so that, for instance, drinking becomes more an everyday activity instead of being concentrated on special occasions and weekends. Finally, the nature of drinking contexts may change, as is happening in the wine-drinking countries where drinking at meals is increasingly replaced by leisure drinking, with intoxication as a crucial element (Pyörälä 1990). A systematic analysis of changes in drinking patterns related to changes in aggregate consumption would require a series of comparable studies over longer periods of time. Such studies are becoming available. As an example, an analysis carried out in Finland (Simpura 1987), showed that in a period of rising consumption from 1968 to 1976, there was first a rise in drinking frequency, and later a decrease in abstinence rates which contributed to consumption growth. In a later period of stable consumption (from 1976 to 1984), changes in abstinence, drinking frequency and intake per occasion, remained small.

2.4 The role of different sectors of the population as contributing to changes in aggregate consumption

Few data are available to allow comparison of changes in consumption of specific population subgroups. Data on trends are mostly available only in relation to the gender variable. In the 1980s, women's share of aggregate alcohol consumption in industrialized countries was stable at roughly 25–30%. Radical changes in the shares of men and women have only been reported in connection with large reforms in alcohol sales and control policies, such as occurred in Finland in 1968 (Simpura 1987). As comparable longitudinal data sets on drinking patterns become available (Fillmore *et al.* 1991), more detailed analyses of the contribution of population subgroups to changes in aggregate alcohol consumption should in the near future be possible. In general, the experience so far suggests that the relative consumption of different sectors within a population are likely to be fairly stable over relatively short periods of time, although longer periods may produce more radical differential movement.

2.5 A multitude of trends

The international picture of trends in aggregate alcohol consumption suggests a diversity in patterns of change – the world is not at present moving in any one drinking direction. In traditional wine countries, consumption continues to decrease, and this decreasing trend has been seen in a number of other Western industrialized countries. In yet other industrialized countries, alcohol consumption continues to increase. In particular, many central and eastern European countries are facing a disturbing growth in drinking and drinking problems. In some areas of the developing world, the consumption of commercially produced beverages is growing, but although monitoring of consumption would be highly relevant to national health planning, reliable data are not usually available. Accompanying the changes in overall consumption are changes in beverage choice, changes in drinking patterns, and sometimes also a new division of consumption between population subgroups. Across the world and in relation to all these dimensions, there are instances of rapid flux, slow change, or steady state. The one firm overall conclusion to be drawn for any country must be, as we said earlier, that levels and patterns of drinking are not set for all time. That fact carries profound implications for health and social policies.

References

Fillmore K., Hartka E., Johnstone B.M., Leino E.V., Motoyoshi M., and Temple M.T. (1991) The collaborative alcohol-related longitudinal project: preliminary results from a meta-analysis of drinking behavior in multiple longitudinal studies. *British Journal of Addiction* **86**, 1203–1210.

Kortteinen T. (1988) *Agricultural Alcohol and Social Changes in the Third World*. Helsinki: Finnish Foundation for Alcohol Studies, Publication No. 38.

Lehto J. and Moskalewicz J. (1994) *Alcohol policy during extensive socio-economic change*. Copenhagen: WHO Regional Office for Europe.

Mäkelä K., Room R., Single E., Sulkunen P., Walsh B., Bunce R, *et al.* (1981) *Alcohol, Society and the State*, Vol. 1. Toronto: Addiction Research Foundation.

Maula J., Lindblad M., and Tigerstedt C. (ed.) (1990) *Alcohol in Developing Countries*. NAD Report 18. Helsinki: Nordic Council for Alcohol and Drug Research.

Negrete J.C. (1980) Sociocultural and economic change in relation to alcohol problems. In: Moser J. (ed.) *Prevention of Alcohol-Related Problems*, pp. 159–170. Toronto: Addiction Research Foundation.

Pyörälä E. (1990) Trends in alcohol consumption in Spain, Portugal, France and Italy from the 1950s until the 1980s. *British Journal of Addiction* **85**, 469–477.

Room R. (1991) Cultural changes in drinking and trends in alcohol problems indicators: recent US experience. In: Clark W.G. and Hilton M.E. (ed.) *Alcohol in America*, pp. 149–162. Albany, NY: SUNY Press.

Simpura J. (ed.) (1987) Finnish Drinking Habits. Results from Surveys Held in 1968, 1976 and 1984. Helsinki: Finnish Foundation for Alcohol Studies.

Smart R.G. (1991) World trends in alcohol consumption. *World Health Forum* **12**, 99–103.

Spring J.A. and Buss D.H. (1977) Three centuries of alcohol in Britain. *Nature* **270**, 567–572.

Sulkunen P. (1976) Drinking patterns and the level of alcohol consumption: an international overview. In: Gibbins R.J., Israel Y., Kalant H., Popham R.E., Schmidt W., and Smart R.G. (ed.) *Research Advances in Alcohol and Drug Problems*, pp. 223–281. New York: John Wiley.

Sulkunen P. (1983) Alcohol consumption and the transformation of living conditions. A comparative study, pp.247–297 In: R.G. Smart, F.B. Glaser, Y.Israel, H. Kalant, R.E. Popham and W. Schmidt (eds.) *Research Advances in Alcohol and Drug Problems, Vol. 7*, New York: Plenum.

Walsh, B. and Grant, M. (1985) *Public Health Implications of Alcohol Production and Trade*. WHO Offset Publication No. 88. WHO: Geneva.

Wilson G.B. (1940) *Alcohol and the Nation*. London: Nicholson and Watson.

World Drink Trends (1992). Produktschap voor Gedistilleerde Dranken, and NTC Publications, Henley-on-Thames.

3

The individual's drinking and degree of risk

This chapter will examine a variety of questions relating to the individual's drinking and degree of risk. The starting point for such discussions must be a sympathetic awareness of the real-world dilemma which confronts every drinker: alcohol can cause both pleasure and pain, but what is the *likelihood*, either immediate or remote, of a given quantity or pattern of drinking leading to positive or negative consequences? If that is a personal question for the individual, the relevant answers must, of course, also be significant in their bearing on public policy. The scientific understanding of individual risk, which is the focus of the present chapter, is highly important to an understanding of population level risk (the concerns of Chapter 4).

The chapter begins with a consideration of 'the drinker's dilemma' – the difficult calculus of individual decision making. In Sections 3.2 and 3.3 a close look will be taken at the concept of *risk curve* as applied to relationships between drinking levels and consequent problems. Matters relating to the interpretability of the relevant evidence will be critically examined. Only with those background matters carefully scrutinized will the chapter go on to present the research evidence on the relationship between drinking and a range of positive and negative consequences, including the relation with physical illnesses, with accidents and violence, with adverse social consequences, with alcohol dependence, and finally with all-cause mortality (3.4–3.10). In some of these areas the research evidence is still scanty, while in other sectors the evidence on the risk functions is substantial and persuasive. The chapter at the end comes back to the question of how all these data bear on practical issues and the public health message (3.11).

3.1 The drinker's dilemma

Alcohol can bring both positive and negative consequences for the individual. These effects can occur in the short- or long-term. Thus a given drinking occasion may provide immediate gratification through alcohol's effect as a mood modifier, as an anodyne or intoxicant, or as a facilitator of sociability. Conversely, the drinking occasion may bring with it conflict, injury, or social opprobrium. At the other extreme, a drinking occasion can make a small contribution to a death from cancer many years later.

Some effects of drinking are relatively certain. For a given level of intake, an experienced drinker may be able to predict with precision what alteration in mood will result, and what extent of hangover will be experienced the next morning. But most effects of drinking are more probabilistic. Only a minority of chronic heavy drinkers die from the long-term physical consequences of alcohol consumption, and the chances of being injured or killed on any particular occasion of drinking and driving are quite small. For some effects, the drinker may have had no personal knowledge of anyone who has experienced the effect, so that the possibility remains rather abstract.

Society often tends to assume that a drinker (at least a drinker who is not dependent on alcohol), will weigh all these possible or probable outcomes against each other in a decision process about drinking: on balance, does the likelihood of pleasure outweigh the likelihood of pain? We may expect different drinkers to evaluate differently how much present pleasure there must be to balance the 'sermons and soda-water the day after'. Presumably the balance will change for each succeeding drink in a drinking occasion, until the drinker stops drinking when the expected balance tips to the negative side. This assumes that the drinker's level of intoxication does not affect the capability to make a rational choice.

So far, we have considered only the effects of drinking on the individual drinker. But drinking also often carries with it effects on others than the drinker – in the economist's jargon, 'externalities'. A drinking driver may cause injury to others; conversely, others may take advantage of an intoxicated person for their own benefit. A drinker may, altruistically or for fear of social sanctions, take some of the externalities into account, but it is unlikely that they will or can all be taken into account.

The dilemma facing the drinker is thus that with each sip he or she faces an impossible burden in calculating and balancing the probabilities of all the possible pleasures and pains. How and to what extent conscious decisions are actually made about potentially risky behaviours is an important current topic of research. Here it suffices to say that a rigid individual utilitarian or rational-choice model is not an adequate account of actual drinking behaviour.

3.2 A risk-curve approach to individual benefit and harm

In this chapter the focus will be on the risk curve associated with a particular aspect of drinking for a particular health or social benefit, or problem. Our primary emphasis is on consequences which are important both in their seriousness and in their prevalence rate. Is there a threshold level of drinking below which there is no association of the drinking level with the consequence? Is there a J-shaped relationship where the relation is actually reversed at lower levels of consumption? Does the risk of the consequence increase more or less proportionately with the rise in consumption, or is the relation curved so that the rate of the consequence rises more steeply at higher consumption levels? These are the kinds of questions which need to be answered in considering risks for the individual drinker. They also, of course, have implications for the relation of drinking levels with consequences at the population level (Chapter 4). And as will again be stressed in Chapter 4, we are not seeking to uncover natural laws or invariable relationships, but rather to describe the general trends which are apparent in the empirical findings. We would caution against any belief that risk relationships array themselves with mathematical exactness along any type of curve, but it is none-the-less robustly true that risks for different types of problems can give rise to risk functions of sharply different form.

There are two specific frames of reference in which these questions have commonly been posed, and in which risk curves for alcohol consumption are commonly presented. One is the literature on alcohol's involvement in chronic mortality and morbidity, where the aspect of alcohol measured is usually a reported drinking pattern at a given time (often interpreted as a surrogate for the cumulative drinking level over time). The other is the literature on alcohol's involvement in casualties, particularly traffic casualties, where the aspect of alcohol measured is usually the blood alcohol concentration (BAC) at a given moment, or some other measure for the level of intoxication at the event. In both literatures, risk curves for a particular consequence of alcohol can be found, often controlling for other factors.

The question of the relation of alcohol consumption to particular consequences arises also in other literature such as studies of alcohol's role in crime or in psychological and social problems. In such literature, however, the approach has often been in terms of summary correlational statistics, often with an emphasis on testing how other variables affect the bivariate relationship by a multivariate analysis. While testing for threshold effects and U-shaped relationships is possible in such analyses, the form of the risk curve for alcohol consumption with respect to the consequence has not usually been a research focus. The lack of interest in risk curves has also sometimes reflected prevailing explanatory beliefs. For instance, at the height of the alcoholism movement, the question of the relation between amount of drinking and alcoholism was rarely asked, since the amount drunk was assumed to be irrelevant to whether someone was an alcoholic (Room 1968; 1983b).

The emphasis on risk curves for alcohol consumption in chronic morbidity and mortality, and in traffic casualties, reflects the importance of measuring 'dose–response' relationships in the two research paradigms respectively underlying these literatures, namely medical epidemiology and behavioural pharmacology. In standard epidemiological discussions of criteria for establishing causality, indeed, the existence of a dose–response relationship figures as an important criterion (Hill 1971).

By itself, a bivariate risk curve linking some aspect of alcohol consumption with a putative consequence, whatever the shape of the curve, is only weak and partial evidence for a causal relationship. Other matters need to be considered in assessing causality, and we will return to this question very shortly (Section 3.3 below). Meanwhile it is worth noting that the raw bivariate risk curve, without controlling for other variables, is of significance in public health programming. A high-risk population subgroup may appropriately be targeted for educational efforts, for instance, irrespective of causation. Thus heavy drinkers might be an appropriate group to warn of the risks of alcohol dependence, even if dependence was seen as caused partially by pre-existing genetic or developmental factors. A bivariate risk curve also matches the form in which advice to the population at large on risks of drinking or on low-risk patterns of drinking is typically given, without differentiation (except often for gender) by demographic and other subgroups of the population.

3.3 Problems of inference from risk curves for alcohol consumption

The existence of a consistent bivariate relationship in a number of studies, particularly when diverse methodologies are used, raises the issue of whether a causal relationship is being measured. However, it by no means settles the matter; attention is required also to other criteria for causality (Hill 1971). In considering the relation of alcohol consumption to putative consequences, there are a number of specific issues which need to be taken into account (Ferrence 1994).

3.3.1 *Failure to measure or classify alcohol consumption appropriately*

The aspects of alcohol conventionally measured in the medical epidemiological and traffic casualty literature only catch the most obvious part of alcohol's potential contribution. For instance, measuring the BAC at the time of committing suicide does not reveal much about the potential causal role of chronic drinking over the longer term. Likewise, a cumulative measure of drinking may not catch the potential role of particular episodes of intoxication in haemorrhagic stroke. For many consequences, there is reason to pay attention to both the amount of drinking or particular drinking events, and to the accumulation and patterning of alcohol consumption over time. Attention to only one aspect may result in an underestimate of alcohol's contribution.

In particular, most medical epidemiological studies summarize drinking patterns in terms of the single dimension of average intake of alcohol per day or year. It can be argued that this is the most important dimension of drinking for cirrhosis and most other long-term physical consequences of drinking, whereas it has long been recognized that whether and how often a person drinks significant amounts on an occasion, are stronger predictors of social and casualty problems (see Sections 3.7 and 3.8 below). Future research should take more account of the likelihood that for some physical harm, too, the patterning of drinking may make a substantial difference to risk. Since a large proportion of the population drinks relatively modest amounts, careful differentiation of light patterns of drinking is particularly important: whether the risk is the same or not for different levels or patterns will, within this part of the spectrum, affect large numbers of people.

The drinking patterns measured and summarized in epidemiological studies of alcohol and physical disease are usually interpreted as representing the respondent's drinking over a considerable period of time, often years. Direct measurement of such patterns is an extremely difficult task. Individual drinking often varies by day of the week, by season of the year, and by life-stage; furthermore, the variation may be quite irregular. General population longitudinal studies (Temple and Leino 1989; Lazarus *et al.* 1991) have found substantial movement between drinking categories over the longer term. In many industrial countries, patterns of sporadic heavy drinking in young adulthood tend to give way in middle age to drinking which is more regular but with fewer 'spikes' of heavy drinking; this in turn tends to give way to much lighter drinking at older ages. Drinking level at a particular time is thus not a good estimate of the cumulative pattern over decades, which may be the most important aspect of drinking for physical health. To the extent that older respondents reduce their drinking, long-term prospective studies using reports of consumption from younger ages will tend to overestimate cumulative amounts of drinking, and thus may underestimate alcohol's effects.

Typically, what studies on the relation of drinking to morbidity or mortality have actually measured is not the cumulative pattern in the long run, but drinking patterns in a relatively limited time period. As we have noted, this is not a good estimate of drinking over the longer term. Depending on the methods used, it may also not be a good estimate of the volume of drinking even in the shorter term. Questions which focus on a short period of time – often as short as a day or two in nutrition surveys – will result in much misclassification, and even questions about the previous week may miss the drinking of many respondents in cultures where sporadic drinking is common (Simpura, 1988; Room 1990; Duffy and Alanko 1992). The conventional method of asking about 'usual' levels of drinking also results in considerable misclassification, since it fails to measure the less-frequent heavier drinking which often accompanies regular light drinking (Knupfer 1987). These inadequacies in measuring patterns of drinking and summarizing them in analysis (Ferrence *et al.* 1986; Knupfer 1987; Colsher and Wallace 1989; Midanik and Room 1992), are often a reflection of the fact that alcohol is just one of a number of potential risk factors measured, and the questions on drinking are accordingly brief.

The usual effect of measuring only a limited aspect of alcohol consumption, or measuring it only for a limited time period, would be to underestimate the true relationship between alcohol consumption and the consequence. However, it is also possible for a systematic mismeasurement to produce an overestimate of the relationship. A Dutch case–control study provides an example. While most modern studies in the literature have collected their data in circumstances where the response will have no consequences for the respondent, the respondent's self-report of drinking is more problematic where respondents do fear consequences – for instance, in relation to their insurance coverage. Thus the finding of a decrease in downhill ski injuries with increasing alcohol consumption (Bouter 1988), is seen by the study's authors as likely to have been due to a retrospective reporting bias; subjects were questioned about their drinking through an insurance company to which they had submitted an expense claim.

Even with the best available questions, general population survey respondents systematically underestimate volume of current drinking, often by an average of one-half (Midanik 1988). This implies that a given level of mortality or morbidity may actually be associated with a level of drinking as much as twice as high as the reported level.

3.3.2 *Effects from 'healthy subject' selection and pre-existing disease*

The age at which subjects are selected, and the method of selection, may produce misleading findings in studies of the effect of drinking levels on physical health. In most case–control studies, subjects are selected at older ages when they may already have developed alcohol-related conditions. De Labry *et al.* (1992), for example, excluded subjects who had a diagnosis of heart disease, cancer, diabetes, or hypertension. Heavier drinkers would be more likely than abstainers to be excluded at this point, since drinking is associated with most of these diseases, and the remaining drinkers could be healthier and perhaps more resistant to alcohol-related diseases than the abstainers.

Since subjects for prospective studies are usually selected through medical or insurance systems as volunteers or through professional associations, individuals who are in hospital or other institutions or who are in poor health, are generally excluded. In studies that use medical insurance plans for recruitment, unemployed or uninsured individuals are excluded. All of these considerations lead to the selection of subjects who are not only healthier than average, but may be more likely to be healthy if they are drinkers. Apart from its possible effect on the measurement of the aetiological relationship, the exclusion of unhealthy subjects also means that the results cannot be generalized to the population as a whole.

On the other hand, inclusion of subjects with pre-existing disease may also result in a misestimation of the relation of alcohol consumption to a physical disease, since, as noted above, sick respondents may have cut down on their drinking. A methodological comparison of study designs relating alcohol consumption to gallstone formation found that the apparent protective effect could be attributed to a pre-existing reduction in alcohol consumption due to gallstone-related dyspepsia (Thijs *et al*. 1991).

3.3.3 *Confounding by smoking, diet, life-style, and other factors*

Most modern studies of the relation of drinking to physical health make an effort to control for smoking status, but the strong relationship between drinking and smoking can make this difficult. Heavy drinkers who have never smoked are rare, as are heavy smokers who are life-long abstainers.

Diet is an important factor in many diseases. It may be implicated in one-third of all cases of coronary heart disease (CHD) and cancers in the West (USDHHS 1988), and is implicated in hypertension, stroke, diabetes, and obesity. Most studies do not control for diet, although data are often collected; furthermore, the narrow range of dietary habits within most study populations can make controls ineffectual.

More generally, different patterns of drinking may be associated with a variety of life-style factors and behavioural patterns, which could confound the relationship between drinking and a putative consequence. For example, it has been pointed out that lifelong abstention in North America has a variety of consistent correlates. Lifelong abstainers are reported to be older, lower in socio-economic status, to live in rural areas, to be religious, to have relatives with alcohol-related problems (Hughes *et al*. 1985; Wannamethee and Shaper 1988), to have higher depression scores, and to experience more depressive symptoms following life events than light or moderate users (Bell *et al*. 1977; Neff and Husaini 1982). Adjusting for the various covariates of abstention does not necessarily affect the risk of mortality (Camacho *et al*. 1987).

Nevertheless, the possibility that such major clustered differences may not be fully amenable to statistical control needs to be considered (Kozlowski and Ferrence 1990). Even controlling for a single potential confounding factor may have its pitfalls. Where there is a functional relationship between potential risk factors, statistical controls may obscure causal pathways. For instance, if being in a drinking situation is a regular cue for smoking, the drinking indeed potentially has a causal relationship with any harm caused by the smoking, but this relationship will be obscured by controlling out the smoking.

On the other hand, in attempting to control for confounding factors, case–control studies may sometimes eliminate part of the alcohol effect. For instance, a study of casualties which matches drivers involved in accidents to other drivers found at the same place and time, underestimates the effect of drinking if part of the effect is on the decision to drive at a dangerous place and time.

3.3.4 *Limitations of generalizability*

It is important to keep in mind that any bivariate risk curve is conditioned on the special characteristics of the population on which it is based. This is especially obvious for social consequences of drinking. Risk curves for the relation of drinking with criminal violence are likely to reflect culturally-specific relations of drinking with violence (Lenke 1990), and risk curves for the husband or wife complaining about drinking will be affected by cultural rules on gender interactions. Comparing risk curves for the same phenomenon in different cultures and social segments, in fact, is a potential tool for examining deeper patterns of cultural variation.

Less obviously, risk curves for other consequences are also conditioned by the characteristics of the particular population on which they are based. In particular, most risk curves for alcohol's role in chronic diseases are based on populations in industrialized, English-speaking, and northern European societies. Compared with the world average, these societies share a number of characteristics likely to affect the shape of the curves: for instance, a majority of the population drinks alcoholic beverages, the diet is rich in animal fats, and heavy smoking is fairly prevalent. Risk curves for alcohol and morbidity in developing countries might well look different.

3.3.5 *The relation of drinking to the consequence*

Risk curves have classically been used to relate drinking variables to consequences where drinking is neither a necessary nor a sufficient cause. A traffic accident can occur without drinking, as can liver cirrhosis. The risk curves have in fact often been plotted as part of research to establish or test a causal connection at the aggregate level between alcohol consumption and the consequence: other things being equal, consuming alcohol in a given pattern affects the risk of the consequence occurring. Even when the causal connection is established at the aggregate level, this does not mean that alcohol is necessarily involved in what happens in a particular case at the individual level.

This classical kind of analysis can be extended beyond the type of consequences to which it has traditionally been applied, but its application in individual-level studies to consequences such as crime or family disruption raises formidable methodological problems: the potential interactions which bear on causal inferences become very numerous. As we shall discuss, the most persuasive evidence for causality in these areas comes from aggregate-level studies.

There are two main ways in which the relationship between drinking and the consequence can be built into the data. One is by external attribution. Some consequences are alcohol-related by definition; for instance, an arrest for driving under the influence of alcohol. Here the law and the police officer are making the attribution about drinking which defines the nature of the crime. Other external attributions may come from health or social service professionals; for instance, a diagnosis of alcoholic cirrhosis, or of alcohol dependence, or a categorization as homeless alcoholic.

The other main mode of attribution is by the drinker him- or herself. Population surveys have often asked respondents to report their 'experiences related to drinking', including social, psychological, and health consequences. The issue of when and under what circumstances respondents will make such causal attributions is an important research question. At a given level or pattern of drinking, the risk curve reveals that a specific proportion of drinkers has reported the particular adverse or positive experience related to drinking.

In some circumstances, the attribution may combine the drinker's report with professional judgement. It is typically the drinker's report on a list of experiences, for instance, which provides the raw material for a diagnosis of alcohol dependence. But the diagnosis of dependence is then made on the basis of professional judgement, either in person by a professional, or according to professionally determined algorithms in a, diagnostic questionnaire.

It should be noted that the causal attribution which is being made is that a consequence or experience is related to alcohol, not to some particular pattern of drinking. There is no necessary causal connection between a particular pattern of drinking and the alcohol-related consequence against which it is being plotted. Nor is the direction of causation always clear. In particular, the reported drinking behaviour may be as much a consequence as a cause of the phenomena diagnosed as alcohol dependence.

A risk curve for an alcohol-related effect of the kind which we are now discussing thus differs from the usual risk curves for cancer or for traffic crashes. The value of the curve is not necessarily as a test of causation, but rather to offer guidance on the probabilities of a given alcohol-related effect at different levels of drinking.

3.4 Drinking and likelihood of positive social consequences

In recent years, the main focus for discussion of potential positive consequences of drinking has been on the possible role of alcohol in reducing the risk of CHD, an issue to which we will shortly turn. However, most drinking is not primarily motivated by a concern for the heart. Drinking, and the feelings associated with sociable drinking, are a source of pleasure to many. Since the main pharmacological effects of ethanol are as a depressant, drinking has also traditionally been used to affect mood, or as an anodyne.

For non-habituated users, some of the positive consequences of drinking may be attained with rather little alcohol. Indeed, expectations concerning drinking may produce the positive effects even when there is no alcohol in the drink, since the positive feelings are often as much a matter of the occasion and the company, as of the ethanol (Lang 1983). However, in general population surveys heavier drinkers report more positive effects of drinking than lighter drinkers (Hauge and Irgens-Jensen 1990). This does not mean that lighter drinkers would report the same level of positive effects if they drank more; there is probably a selective effect at work, where those who receive more positive effects are more likely to become heavier drinkers.

The positive consequences of drinking for the individual are often discussed in terms of an idealized picture of friends sharing a glass or two of wine over dinner. However, Hauge and Irgens-Jensen (1990) found that reported positive effects were more strongly related to the frequency of intoxication than to total volume of consumption. This study was reporting on four Scandinavian societies where intoxication has been the traditional style of heavy consumption, and results might well differ in Mediterranean countries, for instance. Using the Finnish data from the same study, Mäkelä and Mustonen (1988) showed that the experienced positive effects of drinking increased more slowly with increasing consumption than adverse social and official reactions to drinking. For the individual drinker, the ratio of positive to negative consequences thus tended to diminish with higher levels of drinking; the highest ratio of positive to negative consequences was among respondents reporting consumption in the range of one to four drinks per day.

Studies plotting probability curves for positive psychological and social effects of drinking remain few; Mäkelä and Mustonen's approach of comparing risk curves for positive and negative effects should be replicated in other populations.

3.5 Drinking and likelihood of positive physical consequences

3.5.1 *Coronary heart disease*

In a number of studies, drinking one to two drinks per day (but ranging from occasional drinking up to six drinks per day), appears to offer a health benefit compared with lifelong abstention. Among relevant reports and reviews are Klatsky *et al*. 1981; Marmot 1984; Friedman and Kimball 1986; Shaper 1990, 1993; Marmot *et al*. 1981; Beaglehole and Jackson 1992; Kemp 1993; Stampfer *et al*. 1993; Anderson 1994. There is more abundant evidence for men than for women, but the relationship seems to hold for both genders. While this literature can be criticized on many of the methodological grounds discussed in 3.3 above, the provisional conclusion to be drawn is that drinking modest amounts of alcoholic beverages is likely to reduce the risk of CHD for some populations. In Figure 3.1 results are presented graphically from seven studies which showed a negative relationship between drinking and CHD mortality for men. In all seven studies, adjusted relative risks are presented. Different reports have adjusted for different variables, but all have done so at least for age and smoking.

The search for biological mechanisms to explain the reduced risk for CHD and some types of cardiovascular disease (CVD) is active, but has not so far been entirely successful. Most efforts have focused on lipid levels and platelet aggregation (Rankin 1994). Alcohol consumption increases high-density and decreases low-density lipoproteins (Arria and Van Thiel 1992; Rankin 1994; Renaud *et al*. 1993). In the American Lipid Research Center Study and the Honolulu Heart Study, about half the association between non-drinking and CHD could be accounted for statistically by the lower concentrations of high-density lipoprotein cholesterol. It has been suggested that some of these effects are limited to genetically specific subgroups of the population. Alcohol may also act more immediately to reduce the risk of a heart attack by reducing the clotting activity of blood (Zakhari 1991; Rankin 1994).

In the light of the epidemiological literature, it is possible to specify some of the parameters of any such reduction in risk:

1. The greatest part of the reduction in relative risk compared with abstention occurs at very light patterns of drinking, such as one drink every second day, up to about two drinks per day. Any further

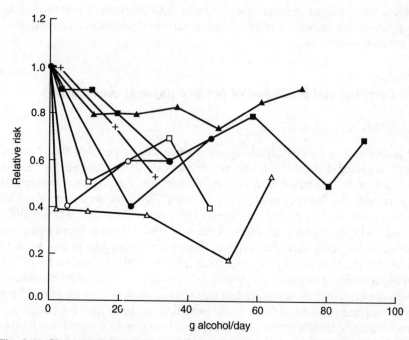

Fig. 3.1. Coronary heart disease mortality among men: alcohol consumption and relative risk. Results from seven studies. Hennekens *et al.* (1978), •; Rimm *et al.* (1991), +; Gordon and Kannel (1983), ■; Gordon and Doyle (1987), □; Boffeta and Garfinkel (1990), ▲; Scragg *et al.* (1987), ○; Jackson *et al.* (1991), △.

reduction in CHD risk achieved beyond that level of drinking is likely to be outweighed by increased risk of other adverse consequences.

2. In particular, a pattern of weekend heavy drinking, which might correspond to an average of two or three drinks a day, carries risks for physical health as well as social and casualty consequences, while it is uncertain whether such concentrated drinking would reduce the risk from CHD.

3. The choice of alcoholic beverage does not appear to affect the reduction in risk.

4. There are no substantial reductions in absolute risk from light drinking for men under 35 and for premenopausal women, since CHD is not an important cause of mortality for these categories, unless it is assumed that a significant later protection will build up from earlier consumption.

5. For those with behavioural patterns associated with reduced risk of CHD (non-smokers who engage in physical activity and eat a low-fat diet), light drinking is unlikely to offer much added reduction in absolute risk. Due to the low-risk behavioural patterns in some cultures, particularly in some developing societies, CHD is essentially unknown; in these circumstances, light alcohol consumption cannot offer a reduction in absolute risk.

6. It is likely that the reduction in risk from light drinking can also be attained by other means, for example, avoiding tobacco smoke, engaging in physical activity, eating a low-fat diet or taking half an aspirin every other day (*Drugs and Therapeutics Bulletin* 1994). Those with reason to avoid drinking thus have other options to reduce their risk of CHD.

3.5.2 *Other positive physical consequences*

Besides the literature on CHD, there are some reports of modest amounts of drinking reducing the risk of other health problems (Colsher and Wallace 1989; Poikolainen 1994). The strongest evidence, for ischaemic but not haemorrhagic stroke, is noted below. In relation to certain other protective effects the seemingly positive findings may have been artefactual (Bouter 1988, Thijs *et al.* 1991, see above).

3.6 Drinking and the likelihood of negative physical consequences

Heavy drinking increases the risk of morbidity and mortality, and the risk rises with an increase in the level of drinking. Our understanding of what lies behind this statement has been enriched by the work of the last 20 years. On the one hand, much of the evidence we have just reviewed showing that modest amounts of drinking may lower the risk of CHD has accumulated in that period. On the other hand, the same decades have seen the list of health conditions in which drinking is implicated lengthened, and the strength of the evidence on the causal effects of drinking increased. In summarizing this evidence, we draw here particularly on recent reviews of the relevant literature (J.C Duffy 1992; Anderson *et al.* 1993; Anderson 1994).

It remains true that we have much stronger epidemiological evidence for mortality than for morbidity. For this reason, our focus here is primarily on increased mortality associated with drinking. It should be recognized, however, that drinking is implicated in a great deal of illness that does not result in death.

3.6.1 *Malignancies*

A review panel of the International Agency for Research on Cancer (IARC; 1988) concluded that alcohol is causally related to cancers of the mouth, pharynx, larynx, oesophagus, and liver. There is a dose–response relationship in most studies after controlling for potential confounders like tobacco smoking, and the relations appear to hold for women as well as men. The relationship is not a straight line, but shows upward curvature at higher drinking levels (S.W. Duffy and Sharples 1992). Rothman (1980) has estimated that, through its contribution to these cancers, alcohol accounts for about 3% per cent of all cancers in the USA. In countries with other patterns of cancer prevalence that figure is likely to be different.

The last few years have seen the publication of a number of studies of alcohol and breast cancer in women. Evidence is accumulating of a dose–response relationship (see Figure 3.2), with the risk rising relatively slowly but steadily with increasing alcohol consumption. There is some

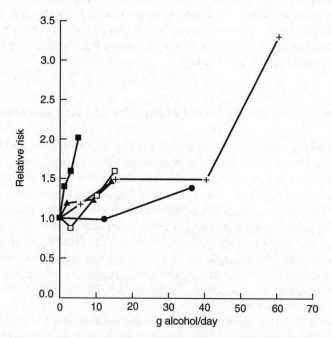

Fig. 3.2. Breast cancer mortality among women: alcohol consumption and relative risk. Five prospective studies. Hiatt and Bawol (1984), •; Hiatt *et al.* (1988), +; Schatzkin *et al.* (1987), ■ Willett *et al.* (1987), □; Gatspur *et al.* (1992), ▲.

variation in results and the relative risks are small, although similar in size to many of the established risk factors for cancer (Kelsey 1993) and opinion remains divided on whether a causal relationship has been established (Hunter and Willett 1993; McPherson *et al.* 1993; Rosenberg *et al.* 1993). Relative risks have here been adjusted for some of the potentially confounding risk factors. All studies quoted have controlled for body mass index, while Schatzkin *et al.* (1987) and Willett *et al.* (1987) have also controlled for diet. Similarly, there is accumulating evidence of a relatively weak dose–response relationship of drinking with colorectal cancer in both genders, with the effect possibly specific for beer drinking (Longnecker *et al.* 1988; Longnecker 1992; Meyer and White 1993). Longnecker estimates that alcohol potentially accounts through these two sites for another 1% of all cancers in the USA.

3.6.2 *Blood pressure and stroke*

High blood pressure is strongly implicated in stroke, meaning that for this area we can draw both on morbidity and mortality studies. Most studies of men reviewed by Anderson *et al.* (1993) show a dose–response relation between drinking and both diastolic and systolic blood pressure, and about half the studies of women show this relation. For both genders, the evidence is split concerning whether the relation exists only above a threshold level of consumption (Beaglehole and Jackson 1992).

Heavier drinking men are at an increased risk of death from all kinds of stroke (Figure 3.3), a result which probably applies for women also. In all of the studies represented in this figure the relative risks are adjusted for age and smoking, and other than Kono *et al.* (1986) and Boffetta and Garfinkel (1990), there has also been adjustment for blood pressure. Underlying this general result, there are both physiological and epidemiological reasons for believing that the relationship with drinking may differ for different kinds of stroke (Arria and Van Thiel 1992). Thus there appears to be an approximately straight-line relationship between amount of drinking and haemorrhagic stroke at least within a certain sector of the risk curve; on the other hand, there is some evidence of a J-shaped relationship with ischaemic stroke, so that lighter drinking reduces the risk but heavier drinking increases it (Arria and Van Thiel 1992; Beaglehole and Jackson 1992; Anders Anderson *et al.* 1993).

3.6.3 *Cardiac conditions other than CHD*

Heavy drinking is associated with increases in cardiac arrhythmias, cardiomyopathy, and sudden coronary death, though the evidence is

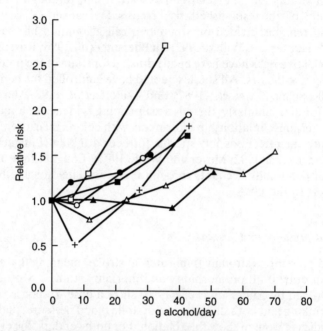

Fig. 3.3. Mortality from stroke among men: alcohol consumption and relative risk. Seven studies. The Kono *et al.* (1986) report subsumed incidence of stroke as well as mortality. Donahue *et al.* (1986), •; Gill *et al.* (1986), +; Kono *et al.* (1986), ■; Semenciw *et al.* (1988), □; Shaper *et al.* (1991) ▲; Ben-Shlomo *et al.* (1992), ○; Boffeta and Garfinkel (1990), △.

still insufficient to determine a dose–response relationship (Anderson *et al*. 1993). Estimates of the proportion of cardiomyopathy cases which can be attributed to alcohol range from 21 to 32%, depending on the samples studied (Arria and Van Thiel 1992). An emergency room study of atrial fibrillation cases under age 65 estimated that drinking was causative or contributory in two-thirds of the cases (Arria and Van Thiel 1992).

3.6.4 *Liver cirrhosis*

The role of alcohol consumption in liver cirrhosis is well established (Smart and Mann 1992). In non-tropical countries with substantial alcohol consumption levels, alcohol is likely to account for upwards of 80% of all cirrhosis deaths (Puffer and Griffith 1967; Schmidt 1977). The dose–response relationship for women appears to be steeper than for men (Anderson *et al*. 1993).

3.6.5 *The shape and steepness of the curves*

Any summary statement concerning the risk curves across such diverse pathologies must be guarded. For liver cirrhosis the relationship may approximate to exponential, whereas for cancers the relationship is more linear, but with an upward curvature at higher drinking levels. For a number of pathologies it would, however, be reasonable to conclude that the risks are increased by between 10 and 30% at a reported consumption level of about 20 g/day for both men and women.

3.7 Drinking, accidents, and violence

Alcohol makes the drinker clumsy, interfering with cognitive, perceptual, and motor skills, and more alcohol makes for greater clumsiness. Thus alcohol is strongly implicated in unintentional injuries and deaths (Romelsjö 1994). Partly because of drinking patterns, and partly because of lesser experience and tolerance, such casualties are especially common among younger adults in many societies, and alcohol-related casualties are a substantial contributor to alcohol-related mortality, particularly when it is expressed in terms of years of life lost. For instance, while it is estimated that alcohol is responsible for 26% of drug-related deaths in Australia (as against 71% for tobacco), it is responsible for 40% of the relevant years of life lost (Pols and Hawks 1992).

There are long-established traditions of research into performance decrement under the influence of alcohol, oriented primarily to aspects of performance relevant to automobile driving, and this literature will be considered again in Chapter 7. In a Report to Congress, the US National Highway Traffic Safety Administration (1992) summarized the effects of relatively light drinking on a variety of performance measures relating to vehicle driving or associated skills. Measurable performance decrements show up even at the level of one drink, although the drinker is often confident that performance has actually improved (Morrow *et al.* 1991). Accordingly (as shown in Figure 3.4), there is no clear threshold to the relationship of blood–alcohol level and traffic crashes. The same is true for associated mortality, with the mortality rising increasingly steeply as blood–alcohol level rises (National Highway Traffic Safety Administration 1992). Although older and more frequent drinkers are somewhat less affected, the relationship remains broadly exponential.

Alcohol is also associated with intentional violence, both towards self and others (Romelsjö 1994). Here the nature of the relationship is more contentious; in addition to psychoactive effects, the link between alcohol

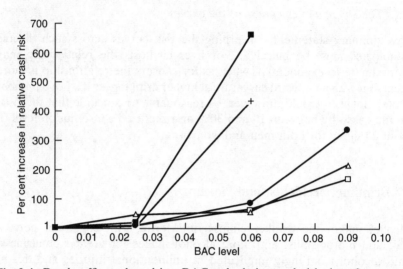

Fig. 3.4. Road traffic crashes: driver BAC and relative crash risk plotted separately for different drinking frequencies. Grand Rapids data, re-analysed. US national data. Yearly, ■; monthly, +; weekly, ●; three times per week, □; daily, △. Source: National Highway Traffic Safety Administration (1992).

and violence reflects culturally formed expectancies about alcohol's effects, and even the excuse-value of drinking. It is generally thought inappropriate to compute relative risk curves for casualties compared with similarly situated non-casualties, as would be done for traffic accidents; it does not seem to make sense, for instance, to compare the BAC of a suicide who has jumped from a bridge with that of someone walking across the same bridge at the same time the next day. The best evidence of causal relations of drinking with suicide, family violence, and other violent crime therefore comes from aggregate-level rather than individual-level data, and thus is discussed in the next chapter (see also Romelsjö 1994).

There is no doubt, however, that level of drinking is strongly associated with engaging in criminal behaviour. In part, this relation is due to alcohol-specific crimes like drinking driving and public drunkenness. Figure 3.5a shows, with data from a large 1988 sample of US adults, that the proportion acknowledging having driven a car in the last year 'after having had too much to drink', starts rising with any drinking at all, and indeed appears to show its steepest rise at levels below one drink a day (Midanik *et al.* 1994). In the same sample, the proportion reporting having been 'arrested or had trouble with the police because of your drinking' in the last year (Figure 3.5b), rose more slowly with volume of drinking, although with no lower threshold for men (Midanik *et al.* 1994).

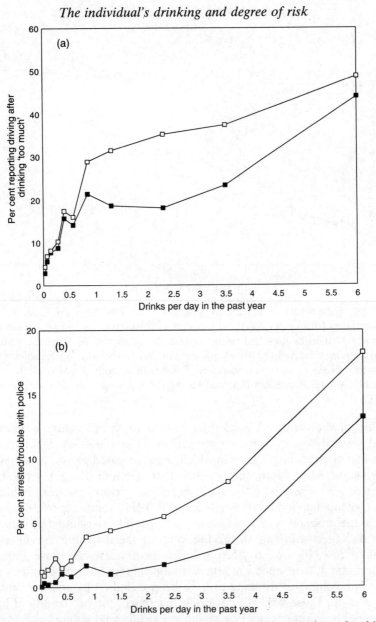

Fig. 3.5 Drink-driving. (a) Alcohol consumption and proportion of subjects reporting having driven during previous 12 months 'after having had too much to drink', with males and females plotted separately. US National Health Interview Survey, 1988. Source: Midanik *et al*. (1994). (b) Arrest or trouble with the police because of drinking. Alcohol consumption and proportion of subjects incurring such trouble during previous 12 months, with males and females plotted separately. Source: Midanik *et al*. (1994). □ males, ■ females.

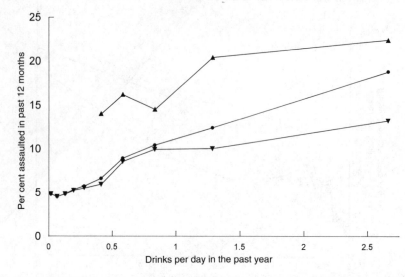

Fig. 3.6. Experience of assault by someone who has been drinking. Alcohol consumption (drinks per day) and percentage of subjects reporting that over the previous 12 months they had been 'pushed, hit or shoved by someone who had been drinking'. Findings plotted separately by frequency with which subjects have consumed five or drinks on an occasion: ▼ less than monthly or not at all; ▲ at least monthly; ● total. Canadian National Survey data. Source: Room *et al.* (1994).

One of the clearest causal relationships in the literature is between drinking and some forms of victimization (Room 1983*a*). Robbery and rape can be predatory crimes in which the intoxicated person becomes the easy victim. More often, the violence arises from drinking in a tavern or other context where both the assailant and the victim have been imbibing. In a Canadian national survey (Room *et al.* 1994), there was a fairly steady rise in the probability of having been 'pushed, hit or assaulted by someone who had been drinking' in the last year, as the respondent's volume of drinking rose (Figure 3.6). Respondents who drank five or more drinks on an occasion at least once a month were much more likely than others with the same volume of drinking to have been assaulted by another drinker; but even for those who did not drink this much, the probability of being assaulted by another drinker rose monotonically with volume of drinking.

The net relation of amount of drinking with death from violence, both accidental and intentional, is stronger than any other relation between drinking and death in many younger populations. For instance, Figure 3.7 shows the relation between volume of drinking and the rates of violent and other deaths, in a sample of Swedish young men followed for 15 years from age 18 and 19.

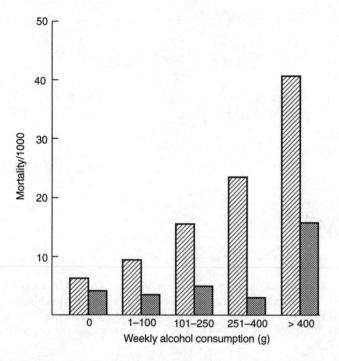

Fig. 3.7. Mortality among young male Swedish military conscripts. Alcohol consumption (g/week) and mortality per 1000 subjects in a 15 year follow-up by violence (▨) and other causes (▨). Source: Andreasson *et al.* (1988).

3.8 Adverse social consequences of drinking

Researchers in the tradition of alcohol social epidemiology have enquired into a wide variety of alcohol-related social problems in general population surveys, including problems with the family, with friendships and at work, financial problems, and arrests and other police problems. Viewed from a sociological perspective, most social consequences of drinking are composed of two elements: a particular drinking or related behaviour, and the reaction of someone else (a family member, a friend, a police officer, a work supervisor, and so on) to the behaviour. Within this perspective, the risk curves may be seen as showing the likelihood that a given drinking behaviour will elicit a particular form of social reaction.

Mäkelä (1978), and Midanik (in press), have reviewed the relationship of drinking patterns to social consequences. The general finding is that the probability of social consequences rises with the level of drinking, however the latter is measured. Figure 3.8 illustrates this with data from a Canadian

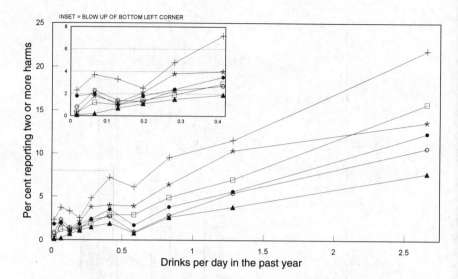

Fig. 3.8. Adverse social consequences from drinking. Alcohol consumption (drinks per day) and experience of harm in six life areas as reported by subjects. Canadian National Survey data. Source: Room *et al.* (1994). Friendships ★; health +; happiness ●; home life ○; work, studies, and employment opportunities ▲; finances □.

national survey of those aged 15 and older (Room *et al.* 1994) in which current drinkers were asked whether they felt that their drinking had had a harmful effect on each of six areas of their life in the previous 12 months. For each life-area, the proportion reporting harm rises fairly steadily with increased volume of drinking, without a clear threshold of amount drunk below which drinkers are exempt from harm. In the sample as a whole, the proportion reporting their drinking had harmed two or more life-areas also rose fairly steadily with volume of drinking (Figure 3.9). A survey of New Zealand adults using the same questions likewise found a roughly straight-line relationship between volume of drinking and the mean number of life-areas in which harm from drinking was reported, although with some levelling off in the harm score at the highest category of drinking volume (Wyllie *et al.* 1993).

In the Canadian sample, at low volumes men were more likely than women to report harm in two or more areas, but above the level of half a drink a day, results were similar for men and women (Figure 3.9). The results for levels above half a drink a day conform to the general finding that women are not more likely than men to report social problems at a given level of drinking. On the other hand, younger adults usually report

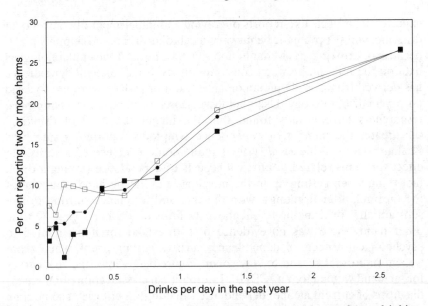

Fig. 3.9. Experience of two or more adverse consequences from drinking. Alcohol consumption (drinks per day) and per cent subjects reporting two or more consequences: □ males; ■ females; ● total. Canadian National Survey data. Source: Room *et al.* (1994).

more social problems than middle-aged respondents for a given level of drinking (Midanik 1994).

As with the results for having been assaulted by a drinker, in the Canadian sample those drinking five or more drinks at a time at least once a month, were much more likely than other drinkers with equal volume to report harm in two or more life-areas (Figure 3.10). Nevertheless, the proportion reporting harm continued to rise with overall volume, among those who did not drink five drinks as often as once a month.

The influence of the context and pattern of drinking on the relation between alcohol consumption and problems must also be taken into account. In line with other evidence on the importance of context of drinking, a recent New Zealand study shows that the amount usually consumed in hotels, taverns, or clubs is more strongly related to alcohol problems than amounts consumed in other locales (Casswell *et al.* 1993).

3.9 Alcohol dependence symptoms

Social epidemiological studies of alcohol problems have routinely included items about physical concomitants of drinking like withdrawal and tolerance, experiential aspects like reports of craving and impairment of control over drinking, and symptomatic behaviours like hiding drinks and skipping meals because of drinking. As Midanik notes (1994), most of the epidemiological data on the relation between consumption levels and alcohol dependence has derived from social epidemiological traditions which were not focused on psychiatric nosology. Using additive scores of dependence symptoms, researchers have usually found that the higher the level of drinking, the greater the number of dependence symptoms reported. Using New Zealand data, Wyllie *et al.* (1993) found some evidence of a threshold effect for items related to physical aspects of dependence (taking a drink first thing when getting up in the morning, and having hands shake a lot the morning after drinking), with the rate and frequency starting to rise substantially for drinking levels above 12 litres of alcohol a year. On the other hand, there was no evidence of a threshold for items related to psychological aspects of dependence, such as getting drunk when there was an important reason to stay sober. Figure 3.11 shows the risk curves for men and women for an ICD-10 (International classification of Diseases) diagnosis of current alcohol dependence (meeting 3+ criteria at some time in the past 12 months), in the 1988 US National Health Interview Survey

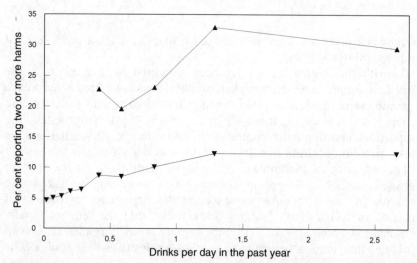

Fig. 3.10. Experience of two or more adverse consequences from drinking, and relationship with pattern of drinking. Alcohol consumption (drinks per day), and per cent subjects reporting two or more consequences, plotted separately for those consuming five or more drinks on one occasion: ▼ less than monthly or not at all; and ▲ at least monthly. Canadian National Survey Data. Source: Room *et al.* (1994).

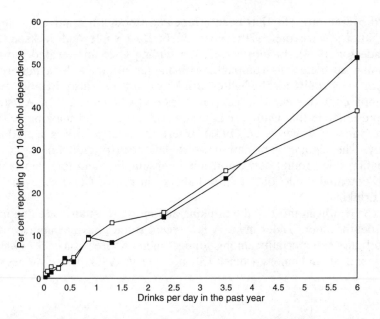

Fig. 3.11. Alcohol dependence. Alcohol consumption (drinks per day) and proportion of subjects reporting symptoms to qualify them for ICD-10 diagnosis of alcohol dependence (3+ criteria met): □ males and ■ females. US National Survey data. Source: Midanik *et al.* (1994).

(Midanik *et al.* 1994). Among both men and women, the proportion with diagnosable dependence rises fairly regularly with level of alcohol consumption. Using the same data, Dawson and Archer (1993) have shown that the proportion meeting a DSM-III-R diagnosis of alcohol dependence (3+ criteria), rises steadily with overall volume of drinking, but for any given volume of drinking is also strongly related to the proportion of occasions at which five or more drinks are consumed. These additive effects remained strong after controlling for demographics, family history of alcohol problems, and age at first drink.

3.10 Individual drinking level and overall mortality

There is no doubt that relatively heavy drinking of alcohol has a substantial adverse effect on physical health. But rather than the sum of all these risks resulting in a straight-line relationship between the individual's level of drinking and mortality, a J-curve relationship between alcohol consumption and overall mortality has been a repeated (though not universal) finding in studies since the 1920s (Pearl 1926; Beaglehole and Jackson 1992; Anderson 1994). In most cases, the finding is of an elevated mortality among abstainers as compared with lighter drinkers. In a minority of studies, mortality for the lightest drinking category is also slightly elevated compared with somewhat heavier drinkers (see Figure 3.12). All studies represented in that figure are adjusted both for age and smoking, with the exception of Kagan *et al.* (1981), where the relative risk is age adjusted only. The leading explanation which has been offered for the J-curve relation often found between alcohol consumption and total mortality, is the potential reduction, discussed above, in risk of CHD at lower levels of drinking.

The deaths in most of the drinking and mortality studies are dominated by deaths among older men. A few recent studies have examined risk of morbidity and mortality among younger men (Andréasson *et al.*, 1988; see Figure 3.7), and among women (Stampfer *et al.* 1988). These studies show

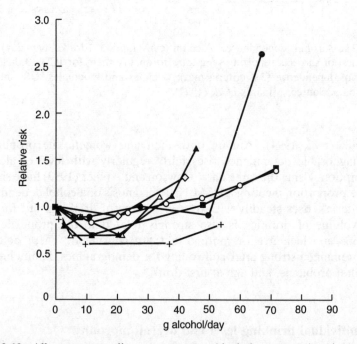

Fig. 3.12. All cause mortality among men. Alcohol consumption (g/day) and relative risk. Eight prospective studies. Dyer *et al.* (1980), ● Shaper *et al.* (1988), +; Kagan *et al.* (1981), ▲; Klatsky *et al.* (1981), ■; Kono *et al.* (1986), ◇; Marmot *et al.* (1982), △; Boffeta and Garfinkel (1990), ○.

a slight but always statistically significant positive relationship between alcohol consumption and overall mortality. In most but not all of the studies that partitioned the total mortality into specific causes, there was a reduced relative risk for deaths from CHD in a band of drinking that extended from a few grams per day to about 40 g/day. Most other causes of death were associated with an increased relative risk of death at all levels of drinking compared with abstainers.

Studies focusing on different sex, ethnic, or socio-economic groups often do not produce the same results as those involving older Western males (Ferrence 1994). The Japanese Physicians Study suggested that relationships between alcohol and total mortality reported in studies of Western populations may not hold for Japanese populations, where the incidence of CHD is much lower and where the incidence of stroke, which is positively related to consumption, is much higher. The British Regional Heart Study reported a protective effect only for smokers and manual workers (see also Kozlowski and Ferrence 1990). As the only large study to look at mortality in younger men, the Swedish Conscripts Study showed no benefit from drinking at younger ages (see Figure 3.7).

3.11 The drinker's dilemma and the overall balance sheet

We noted at the beginning of this chapter that the drinker is faced with an ever more complicated task in balancing the potential for pleasures and pains in choosing to drink, and, for that matter, in choosing to take the next sip. The epidemiological literature can offer little guidance concerning the more experiential side of the pleasures and pains. Concerning more tangible consequences, however, there is some clarity in the picture.

Drinking increases the risk of casualties and social problems, and more drinking increases the risk more. Most of the evidence on casualties and social problems shows no clear lower threshold of risk. From the point of view of these varied and potentially serious problems, the basic message about low-risk drinking is that 'less is better'.

For long-term health consequences, the research reviewed in this chapter confirms a quantitative relationship between drinking and a variety of chronic and life-threatening illnesses, including liver cirrhosis and various forms of cancer. In some instances such as alcohol-related cancers and haemorrhagic stroke there is probably no clear threshold drinking level below which there is no risk.

Evidence has accumulated to suggest that light or moderate drinking can reduce the risk of CHD. Any such reduction must be balanced against the increase of other risks with amount of drinking. It appears that most of the reduction in risk for CHD can be attained with very light or moderate levels of drinking, such as one drink every 2 days. Considering the other social and health risks, such a drinking pattern is therefore likely to be the pattern with the lowest net risk of harm. Most of the reduction in risk of CHD which would be attained by drinking can also be gained by other methods, including regular exercise, a healthy diet, refraining from smoking, and taking an aspirin every second day. Those who choose or are advised to abstain therefore have other methods available to reduce their risk of CHD, as indeed do people who choose to drink. CHD is in any case rare in some developing societies, and in that circumstance the issue of reducing coronary disease risk not salient. In all societies, such disease is not a significant health problem for men under 35 and premenopausal women.

What public health message can come through all this complexity as a sensible message for the individual drinker? Surveys consistently find that regular drinkers substantially underestimate their own consumption, and the pattern of drinking one drink a day and never any more more is rare in societies like the USA (Knupfer 1987). Typically, those who usually have a drink everyday also quite often have more to drink. Any advice to individuals on lower-risk levels of drinking should keep in mind how the advice will play out in the context of existing drinking patterns in the relevant population. We return to policy implications in Chapter 10, where the implications of population (aggregate) drinking levels for public health advice will also need to be taken into account.

The public health message on adult drinking in the modern era has always been complicated; in the terms used for illicit drugs, it is a 'harm-reduction' message rather than a 'just say no' message. The evidence accumulating in the last 20 years has posed the dilemma more sharply, but has not changed the fundamental nature of the problem. On the one hand, we now have evidence for a potential health benefit from drinking in small amounts. On the other hand, measurement of the full range of alcohol-related consequences suggests that entirely risk-free drinking exists only as a fantasy. Prudent advice on lower-risk levels of drinking might therefore set the advised upper limits quite low. What there can be no argument about is that heavier drinking poses very substantial risks, whether the drinking comes in the form of regular consumption at the level of more than a few drinks a day, or of episodes of drinking enough to feel the effects of intoxication. The complexities are real, but the messages that emerge from the evidence which has been reviewed in this chapter are for the individual and society outstandingly clear – less is better, more drinking carries more risk for a wide range of adverse happenings, and heavy drinking is a distinctly dangerous behaviour.

References

Anderson P. (1995). Alcohol and risk. In: Holder H. and Edwards G. (ed.) *Alcohol and Public Policy: Evidence and Issues*. Oxford: Oxford University Press (in press).

Anderson P., Cremona A., Paton A., Turner C., and Wallace P. (1993) The risk of alcohol. *Addiction* **88**, 1493–1508

Andréasson S., Romelsjö A., and Allebeck P. (1988) Alcohol and mortality among young men: longitudinal study of Swedish conscripts. *British Medical Journal* **296**, 1021–1025.

Arria A.M. and Van Thiel D.H. (1992) The epidemiology of alcohol-related chronic disease. *Alcohol Health and Research World* **16**, 209–216.

Beaglehole R. and Jackson R. (1992) Alcohol, cardiovascular diseases and all causes of death: a review of the epidemiological evidence. *Drug and Alcohol Review* **11**, 275–290.

Bell R., Keeley K., and Buhl J. (1977) Psychopathology and life events among alcohol users and nonusers. In: Seixas F. (ed.) *Currents in alcoholism*, Vol. 3, pp. 103–126. New York: Grune and Stratton.

Ben–Shlomo Y., Markowe H., Shipley M. and Marmot M.G. (1992) Stroke risk from alcohol consumption using different control groups. *Stroke* **23**, 1093–1098.

Boffetta P. and Garfinkel L. (1990) Alcohol drinking and mortality among men enrolled in an American Cancer Society prospective study. *Epidemiology* **1**, 342–348.

Bouter L.M. (1988) *Injury Risk in Downhill Skiing: Results from an Etiological Case–Control Study Conducted among Dutch Skiers*. Haarlem: De Vrieseborch, Haarlem, the Netherlands.

Camacho T.C., Kaplan G.A., and Cohen R.D. (1987) Alcohol consumption and mortality in Alameda County. *Journal of Chronic Diseases* **40**, 229–236.

Casswell S., Zhang J.F., and Wyllie A. (1993) The importance of amount and location of drinking for the experience of alcohol-related problems. *Addiction*, **88**, 1527–1534.

Colsher P.L. and Wallace R.B. (1989) Is modest alcohol consumption better than none at all? An epidemiological assessment. *Annual Review of Public Health* **10**, 201–219.

Dawson D.A. and Archer L.D. (1993) Relative frequency of heavy drinking and the risk of alcohol dependence. *Addiction* **88**, 1509–1518.

De Labry L.O., Glynn R.J., Levenson M.R., Hermos J.A., LoCastro J.S., and Vokonas P.S. (1992) Alcohol consumption and mortality in an American male population: recovering the U-shaped curve – findings from the Normative Aging Study. *Journal of Studies on Alcohol* **53**, 25–32.

Donahue R.P., Abbott R.D., Reed D.M., and Yano K. (1986) Alcohol and haemorrhagic stroke. The Honolulu Heart Program. *Journal of the American Medical Association* **255**, 2311–2314.

Drugs and Therapeutics Bulletin (1994) Aspirin to prevent heart attack or stroke. *Drugs and Therapeutics Bulletin* **32**, 1–3.

Duffy J.C. (ed.) (1992) *Alcohol and illness: The Epidemiological Viewpoint*. Edinburgh University Press.

Duffy J.C. and Alanko T. (1992) Self-reported consumption measures in sample surveys: a simulation study of alcohol consumption. *Journal of Official Statistics*, **8**, 327–50.

Duffy S.W. and Sharples L.D. (1992) Alcohol and cancer risk. In: Duffy J.C. (ed.) *Alcohol and Illness*, pp. 1–18. Edinburgh University Press.

Dyer A.R., Stamler J., Paul O., Lepper M., Shekelle R.B., Mckean H., and Garside D. (1980) Alcohol consumption and 17-year mortality in the Chicago Western Electric Company study. *Preventive Medicine* **9**, 78–90.

Ferrence R.G. (1995) Moderate drinking and public health. In: Holder H. and Edwards G. (ed.) *Alcohol and Public Policy: Evidence and Issues*. Oxford: Oxford University Press (in press).

Ferrence R.G., Truscott S., and Whitehead P.C. (1986) Drinking and coronary heart disease: findings, issues, and public health policy. *Journal of Studies on Alcohol* **47**, 394–408.

Friedman L.A. and Kimball A.W. (1986) Coronary heart disease mortality and alcohol consumption in Framingham. *American Journal of Epidemiology* **124**, 481–489.

Gatspur S.M., Potter J.D., Sellers T.A., and Folsom A.R. (1992) Increased risk of breast cancer with alcohol consumption in postmenopausal women. *American Journal of Epidemiology* **136**, 1221–1231.

Gill J.S., Zzezulka A.V., Shipley M.J., and Beevers D.G. (1986) Stroke and alcohol consumption. *New England Journal of Medicine* **315**, 1041–1046.

Gordon T. and Doyle J. (1987) Drinking and mortality. *American Journal of Epidemiology* **125**, 263–270.

Gordon T. and Kannel W.B. (1983) Drinking habits and cardiovascular disease: the Framingham Study. *American Heart Journal* **105**, 667–673.

Hauge R. and Irgens-Jensen O. (1990) The experiencing of positive consequences of drinking in four Scandinavian countries. *British Journal of Addiction* **85**, 645–653.

Hennekens C.H., Rosner B., and Cole D.S. (1978) Daily alcohol consumption and fatal coronary heart disease. *American Journal of Epidemiology* **107**, 196–200.

Hiatt R.A. and Bawol R.D. (1984) Alcohol beverage consumption and breast cancer incidence. *American Journal of Epidemiology* **120**, 676–683.

Hiatt R.A., Klatsky A.L., and Armstrong M.A. (1988) Alcohol consumption and the risk of breast cancer in prepaid health plan. *Cancer Research* **48**, 2284–2287.

Hill A.B. (1971) *Principles of Medical Statistics*, 9th edn. Oxford University Press.

Hughes J., Stewart, M., and Barraclough B. (1985) Why teetotalers abstain. *British Journal of Psychiatry* **146**, 204–208.

Hunter D.J. and Willett W.C. (1993) Diet, body size and breast cancer. *Epidemiologic Reviews* **15**, 110–132.

IARC (1988) *Alcohol Drinking*. IARC Monographs on the Evaluation of Carcinogenic Risks to Humans. Lyons: IARC.

Jackson R., Scragg R., and Beaglehole R. (1991) Alcohol consumption and risk of coronary heart disease. *British Medical Journal* **303**, 211–216.

Kagan A., Yano K., Rhoads G., and McGee D.L. (1981) Alcohol and cardiovascular disease: the Hawaian Experience. *Circulation* **64** (Suppl. III), 27–31.

Kelsey J.L. (1993) Breast cancer epidemiology: summary and future directions. *Epidemiologic Reviews* **15**, 256–263.

Kemp J. (1993) Alcohol and heart disease: the implications of the U-shaped curve. *British Medical Journal* **307**, 1372–1373.

Kittner S.J., Garcia-Palmieri M.R., and Costas R. (1983) Alcohol and coronary heart disease in Puerto Rico. *American Journal of Epidemiology* **117**, 538–550.

Klatsky A.L., Friedman G.D., and Siegelaub M.S. (1981) Alcohol and mortality: a 10-year Kaiser-Permanente experience. *Annals of Internal Medicine* **95**, 139–145.

Knupfer G. (1987) Drinking for health: the daily light drinker fiction. *British Journal of Addiction* **82**, 547–555.

Kono S., Ikeda M., Tokudome S., and Nishizume M. (1986) Alcohol and mortality: a cohort study of male Japanese physicians. *International Journal of Epidemiology* **15**, 527–532.

Kozlowski L.T. and Ferrence R.G. (1990) Statistical control in research on alcohol and tobacco: an example from research on alcohol and mortality. *British Journal of Addiction* **85**, 271–278.

Lang A.R. (1983) Drinking and disinhibition: contributions from psychological research. In: Room R. and Collins G. (ed.) *Alcohol and Disinhibition: Nature and Meaning of the Link*, NIAAA Research Monograph No. 12, pp. 48–90. DHHS Publication No. (ADM) 83–1246. Washington DC: USGPO.

Lazarus N.B., Kaplan G.A., Cohen R.D., and Leu D.-J. (1991) Changes in alcohol consumption and risk of death from all causes and from ischaemic heart disease. *British Medical Journal* **303**, 553–556.

Lenke L. (1990) *Alcohol and Criminal Violence: Time Series Analyses in a Comparative Perspective*. Stockholm: Almqvist and Wiksell.

Longnecker M.P. (1992) Alcohol consumption in relation to risk of cancers of the breast and large bowel. *Alcohol Health and Research World* **16**, 223–229.

Longnecker M.P., Berlin J.A. Orza, M.J., and Chalmers T.C. (1988) A meta-analysis of alcohol consumption in relation to risk of breast cancer. *Journal of the American Medical Association* **260**, 652–656.

Mäkelä K. (1978) Levels of consumption and social consequences of drinking, In: Israel Y., Glaser F.B., Kalant H., Popham R.E., Schmidt W., and Smart R.G. (ed.) *Research Advances in Alcohol and Drug Problems* Vol. 4, pp. 303–348. New York: Plenum Press.

Mäkelä K. and Mustonen, H. (1988) Positive and negative experiences related to drinking as a function of annual alcohol intake. *British Journal of Addiction*, **83**, 403–408.

Marmot M.G. (1984) Alcohol consumption and coronary heart disease. *International Journal of Epidemiology* **13**, 160–167.

Marmot M.G., Rose, G. Shipley, M.J., and Thomas B.J. (1981) Alcohol and mortality: a U-shaped curve. *Lancet* **i**, 580–583.

McPherson K., Engelsman, E., and Conning D. (1993) Breast cancer. In: Verschuren P.M. (ed.) *Health Issues Related to Alcohol Consumption*, pp. 221–244. Washington and Brussels: ILSI Europe.

Meyer F. and White E. (1993) Alcohol and nutrients in relation to colon cancer in middle-aged adults. *American Journal of Epidemiology* **138**, 225–236.

Midanik L.T. (1988) Validity of self-reported alcohol use: a literature review and assessment. *British Journal of Addiction* **83**, 1019–1039.

Midanik L.T. (1995) Alcohol consumption and social consequences, dependence, and positive benefits in general population surveys. In: Holder H. and Edwards G. (ed.) *Alcohol and Public Policy: Evidence and Issues*. Oxford: Oxford University Press (in press).

Midanik L.T. and Room R. (1992) The epidemiology of alcohol consumption. *Alcohol Health and Research World* **16**, 183–190.

Midanik L.T., Tam T.W., Greenfield T.K., and Caetano R. (1994) *Risk functions for alcohol-related problems in a 1988 US national sample*. Working Paper. Berkeley, CA: Alcohol Research Group.

Morrow D., Leirer V., Yesavage J., and Tinklenberg J. (1991) Alcohol, age, and piloting: judgment, mood and actual performance. *International Journal of the Addictions* **26**, 669–683.

National Highway Traffic Safety Administration (1992) *Driving under the influence: A Report to Congress on Alcohol Limits*. Washington, DC: US Department of Transportation.

Neff J.A. and Husaini B.A. (1982) Life events, drinking patterns and depressive symptomatology: the stress-buffering role of alcohol consumption. *Journal of Studies on Alcohol* **43**, 301–318.

Pearl R. (1926) *Alcohol and Longevity*. New York: Alfred A. Knopf.

Poikolainen K. (1994) The other health benefits of moderate alcohol intake. *Contemporary Drug Problems*, forthcoming.

Pols R.G. and Hawks D.V. (1992) *Is there a Safe Level of Daily Consumption of Alcohol for Men and Women? Recommendations Regarding Possible Drinking Behaviour*, 2nd edn. Canberra: Australian Publishing House.

Puffer R. and Griffith G.W. (1967) *Patterns of Urban Mortality*. Scientific Publication No. 151. Washington, DC: Pan American Health Organization.

Rankin J.G. (1994) Biological mechanisms at moderate levels of alcohol consumption that may affect the development, course and/or outcome of coronary heart disease. *Contemporary Drug Problems*, forthcoming.

Renaud S., Criqui M.H. Farchi, G., and Veenstra J. (1993) Alcohol drinking and coronary heart disease. In: Verschuren P.M. (ed.) *Health Issues Related to Alcohol Consumption*, pp. 81–123. Washington and Brussels: ILSI Europe.

Rimm E.B., Giovannucci E.L., Willett W.C., Colditz G.A., Ascherio A., Rosner B., and Stampfer M. (1991) Prospective study of alcohol consumption and risk of coronary disease in men. *Lancet* **338**, 464–468.

Romelsjö A. (1995) The relationship between alcohol consumption and unintentional injury, violence, suicide, and intergenerational effects. In: Holder H. and Edwards G. (ed.) *Alcohol and Public Policy: Evidence and Issues*. Oxford: Oxford University Press (in press).

Room R. (1968) Amount of drinking and alcoholism. Presented at the 28th International Congress on Alcohol and Alcoholism, Washington, DC, 15–20 September.

Room R. (1983*a*) Alcohol and crime: behavioral aspects. In: Kadish S. (ed.) *Encyclopedia of Crime and Justice*, Vol. 1, pp. 35–44. New York: The Free Press.

Room R. (1983*b*) Sociological aspects of the disease concept of alcoholism. *Research Advances in Alcohol and Drug Problems* **7**, 47–91.

Room R. (1990) Measuring alcohol consumption in the US: methods and rationales. In: Kozlowski L., Annis H.M., Cappell H.D., Glaser F.B., Goodstadt M.S., Israel Y., Kalant H., Sellers E.M., and Vingilis E.R. (ed.) *Research Advances in Alcohol and Drug Problems No. 10*, pp. 39–80. New York: Plenum.

Room R., Bondy S., and Ferris J. (1994) *Drinking and Risk of Alcohol-related Harm in a 1989 Canadian National Sample*. Working Paper. Toronto, Ontario: Addiction Research Foundation.

Rosenberg L. Metzger, L.S., and Palmer J.R. (1993) Alcohol consumption and risk of breast cancer: a review of the epidemiologic evidence. *Epidemiologic Reviews* **15**, 133–144.

Rothman K.J. (1980) The proportion of cancer attributable to alcohol consumption. *Preventive Medicine* **9**, 174–179.

Schatzkin A., Jones D.Y., Hoover R.N., Taylor P.R., Brinton I.A., Ziegler, R.G., *et al.* (1987) Alcohol consumption and breast cancer in the epidemiological follow-up study of the first national health and nutrition examination survey. *New England Journal of Medicine* **6**, 1169–1173.

Schmidt W. (1977) The epidemiology of cirrhosis of the liver: a statistical study of mortality data with special reference to Canada. In Fisher M.M. and J.G. Rankin (ed.) *Alcohol and the Liver pp. 1–26. New York: Plenum Press.*

Scragg R., Stewart A., Jackson R., and Beaglehole R. (1987) Alcohol and exercise in myocardial infarction and sudden coronary death in men and women. *American Journal of Epidemiology* **126**, 77–85.

Semenciw R.M., Morrison H.I., Mao Y., Johansen H., Davies J.W., and Wigle D.T. (1988) Major risk factors for cardiovascular disease mortality in adults: result from the Nutrition Canada Cohort. *International Journal of Epidemiology* **17**, 317–324.

Shaper A.G. (1990) Alcohol and mortality: a review of prospective studies. *British Journal of Addiction* **85**, 837–847.

Shaper A.G. (1993) Editorial: alcohol, the heart, and health. *American Journal of Public Health* **83**, 799–801.

Shaper A.G., Wannamethee G., and Walker M. (1988) Alcohol and mortality in British men: explaining the U-shaped curve. *Lancet* **ii**, 1267–1273.

Shaper A.G., Phillips A.N., Pocock S.J., Walker M., and Macfarlane P.W. (1991) Risk factors for stroke in middle-aged British men. *British Medical Journal* **302**, 1111–1115.

Simpura J. (1988) Comparison of indices of alcohol. Consumption in the Finnish 1984 drinking habits survey data. *Drinking and Drug Practices Surveyor* **22**, 3–10.

Smart R.G. and Mann, R.E. (1992) Alcohol and the epidemiology of liver cirrhosis. *Alcohol Health and Research World* **16**, 217–222.

Stampfer M.J., Colditz G.A., Willett W.C. *et al.* (1988) A prospective study of moderate alcohol consumption and the risk of stroke. *New England Journal of Medicine*, **284**, 733–7.

Stampfer M.J., Rimm, E.B., and Walsh D.C. (1993) Commentary: alcohol, the heart, and public policy. *American Journal of Public Health* **83**, 801–804.

Temple M.T. and Leino E.V. (1989) Long-term outcomes of drinking: a 20-year longitudinal study of men. *British Journal of Addiction* **84**, 889–899.

Thijs C., Knipschild, P., and Leffers P. (1991) Does alcohol protect against the formation of gallstones? A demonstration of protopathic bias. *Journal of Clinical Epidemiology* **44**, 941–946.

US Department of Health and Human Services. (1988) *The Surgeon-General's Report on Nutrition and Health*. Rocklin, CA: Prima Publishing and Communications.

Wanamethee G. and Shaper A.G. (1988) Men who do not drink: a report from the British Regional Heart Study. *International Journal of Epidemiology* **17**, 307–316.

Willett W.C., Stampfer M.H. Colditz G.A., Rosner B.A., Hennekens C.H., and Speizer F.E. (1987) Moderate alcohol consumption and the risk of breast cancer. *New England Journal of Medicine* **316**, 1174–1180.

Wyllie A., Casswell S., and Zhang J.F. (1993) *The Relationship between Alcohol Consumption and Alcohol-related Problems: New Zealand Survey Data*. Paper presented at the 19th annual Alcohol Epidemiology Symposium, Kettil Bruun Society for Social and Epidemiological Research on Alcohol, Cracow, Poland, 7–11 June 1993.

Zakhari S. (1991) Vulnerability to cardiac disease. *Recent Developments in Alcoholism* **9**, 225–262.

4

Population drinking and the aggregate risk of alcohol problems

As has been documented in the preceding chapter, alcohol consumption affects people's lives in many different ways. For several diseases there is convincing evidence for dose–response relations between individual consumption and individual risk. Some of these risk functions are strongly non-linear, with more than proportionately greater risk at higher levels of intake. In other cases, J-shaped risk functions have been inferred, particularly in relation to coronary heart disease. And for several types of consequences, the exact relationship between risk and intake is not known, although it is evident that heavy consumption under certain circumstances can elevate risk.

However, from the point of view of prevention, it is not enough to know that excessive drinking often raises individual risk. We also need to know how population problem rates are determined. Population rates of drinking problems vary considerably between cultures and different strata within cultures, as well as within each culture over time (Ledermann 1956; Popham 1970; Mäkelä *et al.* 1981). The aim of the this chapter is to link the individual-level risks to understanding of aggregate-level or population problem rates.

A logical way of approaching the question of population problem rates is in terms of how individual risks vary in response to variation in consumption, and how the population is composed of drinkers with different consumption habits, and hence different risks. One matrix is, as it were, being multiplied into another.

This chapter will therefore be structured in the following way. We will start with a ground-clearing section, which will examine a range of underlying analytical issues relating to the aggregation of individual risks so as to bear on understanding of population problem rates (4.1). What we are seeking to define here and in the following section (4.2), which examines theoretical issues relating to the population distribution of alcohol consumption, is the interactive nature of the function (individual risk from drinking times population drinking distribution), which can be expected to underpin, explain, and predict the later empirical population findings (4.3). We end with a brief preliminary note on the potential follow-through to policy implications. As in Chapter 3, questions relating to the possible protective influence of drinking on coronary heart disease will be examined, but this time at population rather than individual level.

4.1.From individual risks to population risk estimates: analytical issues

4.1.1. *Volume of individual consumption, the shape of the individual risk function, and the prevention paradox.*

In this section we will seek to clarify some important issues relating to the relevance of the shape of the individual risk function for a given type of alcohol-related problem, for population problem experience. For present purposes we will narrow the discussion to situations where cumulative volume of consumption is the major problem determinant, rather than the frequency of drinking large amounts on an occasion.

Intuitively, one might perhaps expect that the population problem rate would be mainly determined by the number of very heavy drinkers. However, this is not necessarily the case, as the contribution of very heavy drinkers to the sum of problems critically depends on how the risk varies with level of intake. This fact underlies the so-called prevention paradox (Rose 1981; Kreitman 1986).

To understand this argument, consider a case where the risk of damage is a linear function of intake (related to intake in straight line fashion). Each extra drink contributes equally to the aggregate problem rate, whether it is consumed by a light drinker or a heavy drinker. Hence, with a linear risk function it does not matter whether everybody drinks exactly the same amount, or if some drink in moderation, while a few drink excessively. The population problem rate would be the same in both cases, and would depend only on the per capita consumption level (Skog 1985a).

Typically, however, the risk for different types of damage is a curved function of intake. The risk is small and increases slowly at low consumption levels, but starts to grow fast at higher levels.

In these latter circumstances and in other than the linear condition, the relative contribution of different consumption groups to the population problem rate is determined by the exact curvature of the risk function. As an illustration, and to render this perhaps at first rather complex proposition readily intelligible, we set out in Table 4.1 two hypothetical and contrasting instances. The population is envisaged as such that 60% drink small amounts, while 35% have a medium consumption level, and the remaining 5% are heavy drinkers. For one type of damage we assume that for the individual the relative risk (RR) increases from 1, to 4, to 20, as one moves from low, to moderate, to high consumption. In that case,

Table 4.1. Relative risks and contribution to overall problem rate, of different consumption groups for two hypothetical drinking problems (60, 35, and 5% of the population are assumed to have low, medium, and high consumption levels, respectively)

Consumption level	Problem no. 1		Problem no. 2	
	Relative risk	% of all problems	Relative risk	% of all problems
Low	1	20	1	9
Medium	4	47	4	20
High	20	33	100	71
Sum		100		100

one-third of the overall problem rate would come from the heavy drinkers, while nearly one-half (47%) would come from the moderate drinkers. For the second type of damage, we assume that the (relative) risk increases much more steeply at high levels, namely from 1, to 4, to 100. In this case the heavy drinkers would contribute most of the problems (71%), while moderate drinkers would be responsible for only one-fifth. The latter case would be representative of chronic diseases following long-term heavy drinking, such as cirrhosis of the liver (Pequignot *et al.* 1978), while the former case may be more representative of certain types of social and acute problems (Moore and Gerstein 1981; Skog 1985*a*, Kreitman 1986).

Hence, at population levels, the relative importance of different groups of consumers for their contribution to the overall sum of damage will tend to vary across types of drinking problems, depending on how the risk function behaves. One cannot always presume that the very heavy drinkers should be the main target for prevention. However, neither should we assume that the prevention paradox applies for all types of problems, as some writers have done (Kendell 1987). For instance, it does not apply to alcoholic cirrhosis, where most of the cases are found among very heavy drinkers (Pequignot *et al.* 1978).

Exactly to what extent and for which problems the prevention paradox applies, is still uncertain. The empirical evidence for its validity largely derives from survey data. Selective non-response and biased samples, systematic variations in willingness to admit problems, failure to take into consideration variations in severity of problems, long latency periods, and so on, may have produced biases in one direction or the other. Improved methods will be needed before one can draw more definite conclusions.

4.1.2. *The relevance of the population composition in terms of drinking levels*

In the example given above, we envisaged the population distribution for levels of consumption as being constant, and then examined the effect of varying the relationship between individual drinking level and problem risk. Unless the individual risk is a linear function of consumption, the composition of the population with respect to intake levels will though also have an effect on aggregate problem rates, and this is the question to which we now turn. Two populations with the same per capita consumption may thus have very different problem rates. Many years ago, this fact was noted by Jolliffe and Jellinek (1941) in relation to cirrhosis of the liver, in their discussion of the correlation between mortality rates and per capita consumption levels across US states.

The degree to which population problem rates will be sensitive to differences in the distribution of consumers across consumption levels, will depend on the curvature of the risk function. If the risk function is strongly curved, as with cirrhosis of the liver, substantial differences in problem rates with different distributions of consumers can be expected. This fact is illustrated in Table 4.2. The table demonstrates how cirrhosis mortality rates would vary across three hypothetical populations each of 100 000 individuals. The populations have the same mean consumption level, but different distributions of drinking. The RR is presumed to increase exponentially with individual consumption. As one can see, in population 1, there are no very heavy drinkers, and the overall mortality rate is only 8.2 per 100 000 inhabitants. In population 2, which has a long tail of drinkers at higher consumption levels, the mortality rate would be more than three times as high at 26.5. In population 3, which is similar to 2, but has a somewhat larger number of very heavy drinkers, the mortality rate would be even greater (36.3). Hence, even a modest change in the tail of the distribution will have dramatic effects on the mortality rate, when the risk function is exponential.

The conclusion to be drawn from this hypothetical but practically relevant analysis, is that the composition of the drinking population can have an important bearing on the population problem rate. Hence, it is of considerable public health interest to obtain knowledge of the distribution of the population according to consumption levels. The effect that a change in the per capita consumption level of a population will have on problem rates, will depend on how the change in consumption is distributed in the population, and this is particularly true for diseases with a strongly curved risk function. We shall address this issue more closely below, in Section 4.2.

Table 4.2. Mortality for a disease with exponential risk function in three hypothetical populations, differing with respect to distribution of consumers according to level of intake, but with the same per capita consumption level

Consumption	RR	Population no. 1		Population no. 2		Population no. 3	
		No. of persons ('000)	Death rate	No. of persons ('000)	Death rate	No. of persons ('000)	Death rate
0	1	20	0.2	20	0.2	20	0.2
1	4	40	1.6	55	2.2	58	2.3
2	16	40	6.4	15	2.4	11	1.8
3	64	–		6	3.8	6	3.8
4	256	–		3	7.7	3	7.7
5	1024			1	10.2	2	20.5
Sum		100	8.2	100	26.5	100	36.3

4.1.3. *J-shaped risk functions*

As has been pointed out in Chapter 3, at the individual level several studies suggest that alcohol may have beneficial effects at low consumption levels, while the risk of damage increases at higher levels. Hence, the risk function may be J-shaped for certain diseases, for instance coronary heart diseases. A J-shaped risk function implies that there is for the individual some 'optimum' consumption level, where the risk is at a minimum level.

There is an interesting consequent question as to what kind of relationship one would get at the aggregate level, if the individual-level relationship is in fact J-shaped. What would happen to population mortality rates for the disease in question, if the aggregate consumption level increased? This would, of course, to a large extent depend on the distribution of drinking within the population.

If only those who consume less than the 'optimal' level increased their intake, while everybody consuming in excess of the 'optimal' level cut back, the mortality rate for the particular disease must decrease. However, this is not a likely outcome, for it would imply that everybody had the foresight to adjust their intake so as to maximize life expectancy. If people really *are* that concerned with their health, why does anybody today drink to an extent that produces problems? The drinkers who are today drinking to such a level that they endanger their health and social functioning, probably would not suddenly stop doing so if it became established as an indisputable scientific fact that moderate drinking provided some protection against heart disease. On the contrary, one could argue that if a substantial fraction of the population (the light drinkers) started to drink more heavily, then those who already drank above the 'optimum' level might be induced to drink more, since they would find themselves living in a wetter environment, with more opportunities to drink. In the psychological literature on modelling, as well as in the sociological literature on small groups, there is evidence to suggest such a contagion effect (for a review, see Skog 1980*a*).

The idea that one could ever engineer society so that across the whole population suddenly everyone drank at one uniform level pegged at the individually defined 'optimum' is, of course, a highly unrealistic scenario, and estimates of potential benefit based on that kind of conjecture are fictional. Drinking habits vary substantially from one individual to the next, and this would in all probability remain so even if everybody knew for a fact that drinking in moderation could be beneficial. Hence, in a real society, some people will undoubtedly drink less than any 'optimum', while others drink more. Thus, at a mean level equal to the individual 'optimum', population mortality rate will not be reduced by as large an amount as would be suggested by calculations based on the abstract individual risk.

The aggregate-level benefit will therefore be considerably smaller than predicted by analysis restricted to individual-level understanding.

In setting public health policies in the presence of a J-shaped risk function, it is thus crucial to make a distinction between the 'optimum' intake level for the individual and for the population. Due to the long tail of the consumption distribution, it is likely that the 'optimum' consumption level for a population will be considerably lower than the 'optimum' level for an individual. How much lower will depend on the shape of the risk function and on changes in the distribution of alcohol consumption, as the consumption level of the population changes. In not too unrealistic circumstances (proportional changes in consumption), the 'optimum' consumption level for the population could be less than the 'optimum' for an individual drinker by a factor of 3 or even 5 (Skog 1992). This would imply that most Western countries are already consuming in excess of the population 'optimum' level. If this is the case, then an overall increase in intake that is triggered by the prospects of health benefits for light drinkers, could in fact result in an overall increase in the mortality rate. However, as has already been noted, a substantial change in the whole distribution of alcohol could, if it occurred simultaneously, theoretically prevent this from happening.

4.1.4. *Duration of exposure and the time-lag problem*

A simple comparison of per capita consumption trends and trends in mortality, may sometimes be inadequate because the short-term view can underestimate the possible complexity of the long-term and follow-through effect of consumption change on the population's health. Many diseases develop only after long-term heavy drinking. This fact has important implications for the aggregate relationship between drinking, and morbidity and mortality (Skog 1980*b*). The consequence of the long latency at the individual level typically will be a so-called distributed time lag at the aggregate level. The effects of an increase in aggregate consumption and thus in the prevalence of heavy drinking, will be spread over a period of many years. A fraction of the increase in mortality will, however, be visible almost instantaneously or within the first couple of years, although the full effect will not have become apparent until about 20 years or so have elapsed (Skog 1984*a*).

A reservoir effect explains the immediate response. There are always a number of drinkers who consume only slightly less than is needed for them to die from, say, cirrhosis of the liver. However, if their consumption goes up, then their disease develops more rapidly, and they may die from cirrhosis within a short time. Other drinkers will need more time to contract cirrhosis and die of the disease, and are responsible for the longer-term effects.

The rapid response in mortality to a dramatic change in aggregate consumption level was illustrated most convincingly in data from Paris during the Second World War. In 1942, rationing was introduced because of an extreme shortage of alcoholic beverages, and consequently there was a dramatic reduction in alcohol consumption that lasted until 1947. The rations were 0.5–1 litre of wine per week, and per capita consumption may have been reduced by 80% or more during the war. The effect on cirrhosis mortality was equally dramatic. After 1 year, mortality was reduced by more than 50%, and after 5 years it was more than 80% below the 1941 level (Figure 4.1).

A time-lag effect implies that the mortality trend will to some extent lag behind the consumption trend. The effect will be particularly pronounced in cases where consumption has been changing in one direction for a long period, and then suddenly changes in another direction. In this situation one might expect a transition period, during which consumption moves in one direction and mortality rates in the opposite direction. This would occur because the full effect of the first trend would not yet have become visible when the consumption trend changed. An empirical illustration of this kind of situation has been observed in Great Britain, among other countries. During the years 1931–1958, Popham (1970) found a negative correlation ($r = -0.61$) between per capita alcohol consumption,

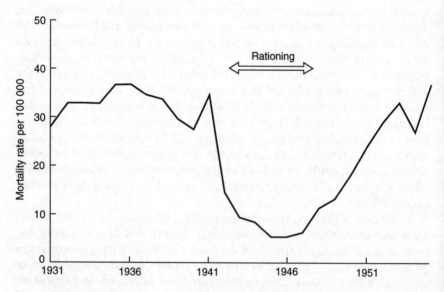

Fig. 4.1. Liver cirrhosis mortality in Paris 1930–1956. (Data from Ledermann 1964).

and liver cirrhosis mortality rates. In all other data sets, Popham found positive correlations. Upon closer analysis, it became apparent that the explanation for the anomaly probably lay in the fact that alcohol consumption had decreased markedly from the turn of the century to the early 1930s. Then followed a period of about 15 years with a moderately increasing trend in consumption, while mortality rates continued to decrease until the early 1940s. When the data were re-analysed, and the distributed time lag taken into consideration, the correlation became positive ($r=0.87$), and well in line with the remaining body of data (Skog 1980*b*).

The time-lag effect clearly needs to be taken into consideration when one evaluates trends in problems following chronic use. Statistical methods for dealing with this have been developed in recent years, and have been applied in alcohol research. Older studies – and even unfortunately some new ones – that fail to take the time lag into consideration may easily produce biased results, and need to be interpreted with care. This problem has become particularly urgent in recent years, since the consumption trends in many countries are no longer uni-directional.

However, in the case of consequences related to acute intoxication, time-lag effects typically do not represent a serious problem. In this situation, confounding in terms of the analysis failing to deal with the interaction between alcohol and other factors, is likely to set the most serious problem.

4.2. The distribution of alcohol consumption

4.2.1. *A historical note*

As we have already argued, the effect of changes in per capita consumption will typically depend on how these changes are distributed in the population. The relevance of this fact was first realized in full by the French demographer Sully Ledermann.

Starting in 1946, Ledermann published a series of studies on secular trends and regional variations in mortality for France and other countries. He observed substantial covariation both in space and time between per capita alcohol consumption and mortality, and this inspired his well-known theory on the distribution of alcohol consumption. Briefly, the theory states that there should be considerable regularity in the way consumers are distributed along the consumption scale, and that this distribution can be approximated by a so-called log-normal probability curve. Moreover, Ledermann presumed that there was a fixed relationship between the mean and the variance of the distribution. The latter relationship implies that changes in the mean consumption level will typically be accompanied by changes at all levels of consumption, including heavy drinking (Ledermann 1956).

Ledermann's distribution theory has caused controversy over the last 25 years, and has stimulated a series of empirical and theoretical studies. The theoretical rationale and empirical validity of the theory's basic hypotheses have rightly been questioned, and it is today generally recognized that the empirical distributions do not have well-defined mathematical properties. Some regularities in distribution patterns have, however, been observed, and these patterns are relevant to the relationship between the overall level of drinking in a society and aggregate problem rates. We shall briefly review two main findings – first, the fact that the distribution is very skew, and second the fact that the prevalence of heavy drinking varies cross-culturally, as well as within each culture over time, with these variations linked to variations in the overall level of consumption.

4.2.2. *The skewness of the distribution*

A priori, the distribution of the population along the consumption scale could have many different potential shapes (Figure 4.2). One possibility would be a uniform distribution (A), with the same number of persons in each consumption interval. A bell-shaped distribution resembling the normal distribution (B) is another possible form, and this is known to apply to some human attributes. A bimodal shape (C) is also conceivable – with 'normal drinkers' at the lower part of the consumption scale and 'alcoholics' more or less clearly separated at higher levels. A fourth alternative would be a skew distribution (D), without any sharp division between normal and 'alcoholic' drinking.

Some of these possibilities can be disregarded on the basis of common knowledge. Symmetrical distributions, like the uniform and the Gaussian, would not allow anyone to drink more than twice as much as the average, since nobody can drink less than zero. We know that in most cultures where alcohol is consumed, there is a significant number of very heavy drinkers, and their intake is substantially higher than twice the average. This argument strongly suggests that the distribution must be asymmetrical and skew to the right (that is, positive skewness).

Many possible additional shapes remain, however. Bimodal distributions may be constructed in lots of different ways, and the class of unimodal, skew distributions is also large. Is it possible to choose a more limited class of distributions on the basis of theoretical arguments or otherwise? Moreover, is it likely that population alcohol consumption obeys any kind of distribution law?

It is known from other branches of life sciences that some human

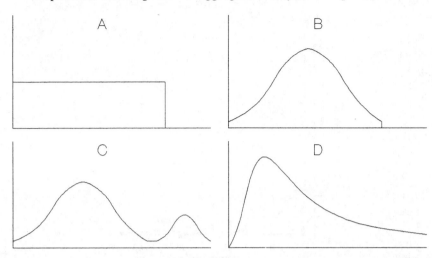

Fig. 4.2. Hypothetical distributions of the population of drinkers according to annual intake.

attributes have distribution laws, at least in an approximate sense (Anastasi 1958). Furthermore, econometricians have demonstrated regularities in the distribution of wealth and income. These distributions are typically very skew and resemble a theoretical curve known as the Pareto distribution (Blinder 1974). Still other examples are known from the study of human consumption behaviour, and consumption of many types of commodities roughly follows a mathematical curve known as the log-normal distribution (Aitchison and Brown 1969), which is unimodal and skew with a long tail towards high consumption levels.

These approximate distribution 'laws' are usually explained by structural features of the mechanisms that determine the attributes in question. For instance, intelligence is typically determined by a large number of different genetic and environmental factors, and all these are assumed to combine additively to produce the overall result.

An individual's alcohol consumption is also determined by a large number of different factors. In this case, however, the factors tend to combine multiplicatively, rather than additively. This has been documented both in cross-sectional and longitudinal data (Skog 1979, 1991), and has the effect of producing a skew distribution, which may resemble the log-normal distribution. However, since some factors have a fairly large impact on consumption, one cannot presume that all factors contribute only a small amount: significant deviations from log-normality may therefore prevail in some populations. This argument is another way of formulating the fact that most natural populations are heterogeneous and consist of different strata

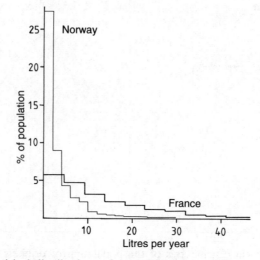

Fig. 4.3. Empirical distributions of annual intake according to surveys in France and Norway.

with substantial differences in mean consumption level. The heterogeneity of populations implies that theoretical distribution laws can only be crude approximations to reality.

That empirical distributions of alcohol consumption are strongly skew, with a long tail towards high consumption levels, is well established. Sometimes the distribution may approximate closely the log-normal curve, while this may not be true in other cases. Two typical examples are reproduced in Figure 4.3, which shows distributions of self-reported alcohol consumption in Norway and France, respectively. As can be seen, there are no clear-cut thresholds separating 'normal' and 'heavy' drinking. In both countries, the majority of the population consumes small to moderate amounts, and as one moves upwards along the consumption scale there is a gradually decreasing number of drinkers. Hence, there seems to be a gradual, rather than abrupt, transition from light to heavy drinkers.

Some writers have suggested that the skewness may be explained by aggregation effects, and that homogeneous substrata could display more symmetrical distributions. This is not correct, however, and even highly homogeneous substrata display very skewed distributions (Skog 1979, 1991). The skewness is mainly due to approximate multiplicativety, resulting from the law of proportionate effects. If one starts with a group of consumers who initially drink exactly the same amount, and follows them over a period of time, one finds that, after some years, they tend to spread out along the consumption scale according to a highly skewed distribution. Moreover, even populations of 'chronic alcoholics' tend to display highly skewed distributions after some time (Popham and Schmidt 1976; Skog and Duckert 1993). And if we look at the distribution of consumers that are not 'alcoholics', we will still be left with a strongly skew distribution. Hence, alcohol dependence cannot altogether explain the skewness. In fact, even non-addictive consumer goods have skewed consumption distributions. Thus, the dependence-producing properties of beverage alcohol may accentuate the skewness of the distribution of alcohol, but are not needed to explain the shape of the distribution.

As was noted above, with a symmetrical distribution, nobody can drink more than twice the average. Hence, the proportion of the population drinking more than twice the average can be used as a measure of the skewness of the distribution. Empirically this proportion is remarkably stable across drinking cultures, and typically varies between 10 and 15% of the population (Skog 1985c). Hence, the tail region contains a substantial number of drinkers.

The strong skewness of the distribution has some important implications for alcohol problems. It means that there is a substantial fraction of the population located at intermediate consumption levels – between 'light' drinking and 'excessive' drinking. From a public health point of view these intermediate drinkers may be a highly relevant sector because the group is large, compared with the 'excessive' drinkers, and this in terms of their contribution to overall population problem experience may compensate for their smaller, but still not negligible risk. One is back here to the prevention paradox.

4.2.3. *The prevalence of heavy drinking.*

A relationship predicted between prevalence of heavy drinking and the overall consumption level in the population is one important inference from the Ledermann theory. Although many other aspects of this theory have not been borne out, the existence of such a relationship has been confirmed by empirical studies. The relationship between population mean consumption per drinker and the prevalence of drinkers with an annual intake exceeding, respectively, 18.75 and 36.5 litres of absolute alcohol, is shown in Figure 4.4. The points in this diagram are empirical observations from population surveys in different countries, while the solid curves are least square regressions. Apparently, the prevalence of heavy drinking, however defined, varies substantially as we go from cultures with a low per capita consumption level to cultures with a high per capita consumption level.

Some writers have claimed that this relationship is tautological, since a high prevalence of heavy drinking implies a high average intake. However, the relationship is of a more profound nature. This has been demonstrated by observing how the distribution changes when one moves from cultures with low to those with high overall intake. This point is illustrated in Figure 4.5, which shows how different percentiles of the distribution change when per capita consumption changes. Low percentiles can be viewed as representing prototypical 'light' drinkers, while high percentiles represent the prototypical 'heavy' drinkers in their respective cultures. Note that 'heavy' here is used in a relative sense, as opposed to the case in Figure 4.4. One observes that, as a rule, all types of drinkers tend to increase their consumption when we move from cultures with low to cultures with higher overall consumption. There is in effect an orchestrated movement of the whole population along the consumption scale. The scales in Figure 4.5 are logarithmic, to bring out relative, rather than absolute, changes.

The patterns observed in Figures 4.4 and 4.5 thus suggest that changes in the general level of consumption in a culture may typically be collective changes across all consumption levels. Some writers (for instance, Duffy 1986) have argued that this conclusion is invalid, since the data are cross-cultural rather than longitudinal. However, several studies of change across time confirm the expectations. Distribution data from Finland, Sweden, Norway, London, and the Netherlands all showed that increasing per capita consumption was the result of a general increase in the intake

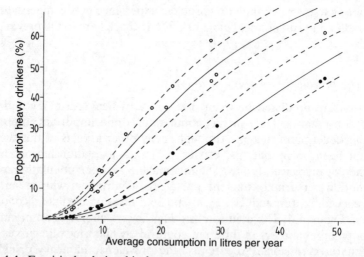

Fig. 4.4. Empirical relationship between mean alcohol consumption per drinker and proportion of population drinking in excess of 18.75 and 36.5 litres respectively of pure alcohol per year. Regression curves (solid curves) and confidence curves (broken curves) are determined by least squares (Source: Skog 1985*c*)

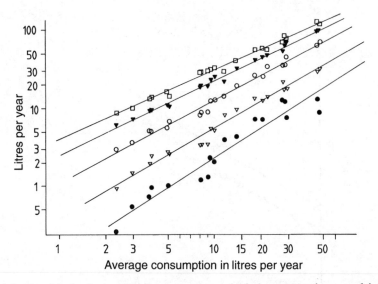

Fig. 4.5. Empirical relationship between mean alcohol consumption per drinker and different percentiles. Straight lines are least square regressions (Source: Skog 1985*c*). Heavy, □; near heavy, ▼; moderate, ○; medium, △; Light, ●.

of all groups of drinkers (Bruun *et al*. 1975. Skog 1985*c*; Lemmens *et al*. 1990).

A typical example is given in Figure 4.6, which shows a log probability diagram (cumulative distributions plot), for Finnish males according to self-reported consumption in 1968 and 1976. The two curves are nearly parallel, and the 1976 curve is shifted to the right of the 1968 curve. This implies that drinkers at all levels have increased their intake to roughly the same extent in percentage terms, and hence that the prevalence of heavy drinking has increased. Using a somewhat different technique, Lemmens *et al*. (1990) demonstrate a similar pattern in the Netherlands.

Although the overall patterns observed in these data are best described by terms like 'collective' differences, and 'orchestrated' change, these descriptions should not be understood in an absolute sense. These statements describe the overall statistical tendencies in the data. We are not proposing a natural law or anything mechanistic and inevitable, and since variations exist around the main tendencies, one should be careful when applying the results to individual country cases. There may be circumstances where changes are 'non-collective', for instance, when some substrata of society increase their overall level of intake, while others decrease, or different strata may change in the same direction

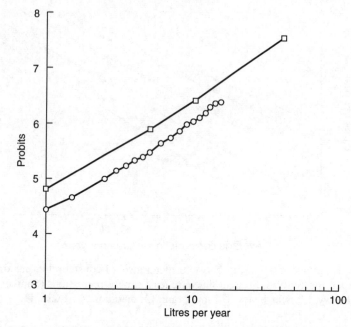

Fig. 4.6. Log probability diagrams for Finnish males 1968 (□) and 1979 (○). (Data from Mäkelä 1969 and Simpura 1985.)

but at highly different rates. Furthermore, the present sociodemographic differentiations of drinking will not remain fixed for all time.

By convention, abstainers are not included in the analyses reviewed above. Hence, mean consumption is calculated per drinker, rather than per capita. One needs therefore to be cautious when applying the results to situations where abstainers are included in the calculations. Whether or not there is a systematic relationship between rates of abstention and the average consumption level per drinker is still not clear. Individual examples of both positive and negative relationships can be found. Given that a change in per capita consumption has occurred, one would ideally like to know to what extent this is due to changes in the abstention rate, and to what degree it results from a change in the consumption level of the drinkers.

4.2.4. *An attempt to explain the observations on population drinking distribution*

When considered as a whole, the data reviewed here suggest that the drinker's risk of becoming a heavy drinker depends on the 'wetness' of the drinking culture to which the person belongs. Environmental factors thus play an important role in the production of drinking problems. It is simply not true that 'alcoholics' are predetermined to heavy drinking, more or less independently of their cultural environment.

The regularities that have been described in the distribution of alcohol consumption can be explained in terms of the socio-cultural genesis of individual drinking patterns. Drinking behaviour is social behaviour in the sense that it is something we learn and practise with other members of our culture. A large number of experimental and observational studies demonstrate that individual drinkers are strongly influenced by the drinking habits in their social network (Skog 1980*a*). The social interaction theory of drinking thus suggest that an individual living in a fairly dry environment may tend to become a light drinker, while the same individual could have become a heavy drinker in a wet environment where alcohol is cheap, easy to come by, and an integral part of daily life. Since individual drinking habits are interconnected through social interaction, individual changes in drinking habits tend to be synchronized, and collective patterns of change tend to follow (Skog 1979). Thus, the collective patterns observed in the data are most probably the products of social and cultural mechanisms.

The apparent absence of a close relationship between abstention rates and drinking levels, may find an explanation within the frame of the social interaction theory. If abstainers and drinkers are only weakly integrated subcultures, changes within the subculture of drinkers may have little impact on the subculture of abstainers. Weak integration may be accounted for by ideological tensions, among other factors.

Typically, the data reviewed describe what one could call 'Western world consumers free markets', with little direct, formal social control of individual drinkers. In societies with much stronger control over each drinker, one could easily imagine that the distribution of consumers according to intake would be quite different. Hence, if formal or informal social controls on individual drinkers were increased, the distribution of consumption would change, and we should expect to see a reduced prevalence of heavy drinking, without a corresponding change in the mean level of consumption (Skog 1980*a*).

Norström (1987*a*) has shown the effect of formal social control on the distribution of alcohol consumption in a study of the so-called Bratt system in Sweden. This was an individual rationing system that was introduced during the First World War (as an alternative to prohibition), and which was in operation until the middle of the 1950s. Norström demonstrated that the rationing system substantially reduced the variance of the distribution and the prevalence of heavy drinking, compared with other countries with a similar mean consumption level. This had substantial effects on liver cirrhosis mortality (Norström 1987*a*), and on crimes of violence

(Lenke 1990). The Swedish case thus illustrates the general point that the regularities observed in distribution data from any country may be modifiable by certain influences or mechanisms, and thus that 'distribution laws' do not apply with unlimited validity.

4.2.5. *Heavy drinking and the nature–nurture problem*

Over recent years the rigid conception of 'alcoholism' as a distinct entity, qualitatively different from normal drinking, has been replaced by the more flexible biaxial concept of 'alcohol dependence' as one dimension, and 'alcohol-related' problems as another (Edwards *et al.* 1977). This conceptual change acknowledges that the condition called 'alcoholism' is many-faceted.

Furthermore, use, misuse, and dependence come in many different degrees, while the transition between so-called 'normal' drinking and 'abnormal' drinking is gradual, rather than abrupt.

This new conception of the issues which are involved is consistent with the perspective outlined here. We have argued that drinking behaviour is influenced by a host of different factors that tend to multiply each other's impact in algebraic fashion. Heavy drinking has a multiplicity of causes, and a heavy drinker is a person who combines a large number of constitutional and environmental 'predisposing' factors, which tend to increase drinking. Each separate factor in itself may not induce heavy drinking. However, the existence of many factors operating in the same direction and amplifying each other by multiplicativety of effects, produces the behaviour. This implies multiple aetiology, and the absence of a clear-cut distinction between normal and abnormal.

The data that have been reviewed here, underline the importance of the environment as a determinant of risk for alcohol problems. This stems particularly from the fact that heavy drinking is closely related to drinking in general. The collective movements of the whole population up and down the consumption scale suggest that normal drinking represents the cultural foundation of heavy drinking, and that the consumption level – and hence the risk of drinking problems – for a drinker with a given constitutional disposition, is directly related to the amount of alcohol to which he or she is exposed in the cultural environment.

This is not a renunciation of the importance of constitutional disposition as a determinant of drinking (Partanen *et al.* 1966; C.C.H. Cook and Gurling 1991; Ball and Murray 1994; Nutt 1994). Whether or not people will become so-called 'chronic alcoholics', depends on their disposition due to constitutional factors – both biological and psychological – as well as the extent to which they are exposed to the agent alcohol. Even people who have a strong constitutional disposition will not become excessive drinkers in the absence of alcohol, or if alcohol is a rare commodity in their environment. On the other hand, even people with a limited constitutional disposition may develop a drinking problem when exposed to a particularly 'wet' environment where alcohol is cheap, easy to come by, and frequently used by everybody. Hence, there is no contradiction in saying that both constitution and the environment are important (Vaillant 1988).

The nature/nurture debate continues and there is much still to be learnt about this interaction as it pertains to drinking behaviour. The point we would like to stress, however, is that our argument remains true irrespective of whether there is a high or low correlation between biological constitution and problem drinking, however construed. Even in the unlikely case of nearly perfect correlation, one would expect the prevalence of 'alcoholics', 'severely dependent drinkers', and so on, to vary considerably in space and time, in response to the variations in the overall 'wetness' of the culture.

The biological factors affecting drinking behaviour are large in number and diverse in nature (Jaffe 1988). No single 'drinking-gene' can be presumed. Some neurotransmitters may affect the pleasures people experience (euphoria), metabolic factors induce aversive reactions to alcohol in some people (Agarwal and Goedde 1991), and a great many biological mechanisms may have more indirect effects on drinking behaviour, by affecting other behavioural dimensions which again influence drinking. Furthermore, these links between genetic make-up and drinking behaviour are certainly not mechanical and inevitable. The presence of such 'predisposing' factors can only produce an elevated *risk* and whether this risk is materialized into a drinking problem, will depend on environmental factors.

Since one must presume a multiplicity of independent genetic factors, genetic disposition ought to exist in degrees, and one can imagine a distribution of the population along a scale that measures 'biological disposition'. Some people have a high, some a moderately large, and some a low disposition. In a low consumption culture, the exposure to alcohol is, on the average, fairly small. Mainly those who have a high disposition would develop a drinking problem in this context. In a 'wet' culture, however, exposure is large, and even those with a fairly moderate disposition may develop a drinking problem (see Figure 4.7). Hence, the prevalence of drinking problems should be larger in the latter case – as available evidence confirms (see Section 4.3 below).

A similar argument may also apply within each culture. Consumption levels and drinking practices vary considerably between different substrata of a population. Clark and Hilton (1991) provide comprehensive US data on this issue), and fairly dry cultures will contain cultural 'pockets' where alcohol is used more freely and frequently. In these subcultures moderately predisposed individuals may be at risk. One would therefore expect that

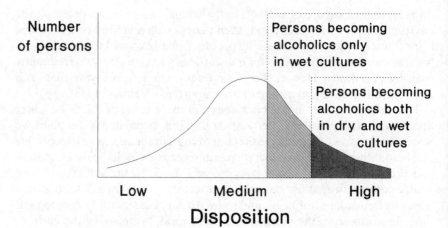

Fig. 4.7. Hypothetical distribution of the population according to disposition for problem drinking.

even rather dry cultures would have a share of 'alcoholics' with a low or moderate disposition, due to the existence of 'wet pockets'. Hence, in any culture, 'alcoholics' are likely to be a fairly heterogeneous group.

4.3. Empirical studies of the aggregate relationship between alcohol and damage

4.3.1. *Non-experimental data: the general need for caution*

The results reviewed in the preceding sections lead one to expect that population rates of alcohol-related problems – particularly the kind of problems where the risk is closely related to the volume of intake – should depend on the overall level of drinking in the population. This proposition is not put forward in a rigid and fixed way, but as a main statistical rule. Below we shall review the empirical evidence for this inference. We start by briefly highlighting some methodological issues that one needs to keep in mind when attempting to test this hypothesis.

Aggregate-level studies of the relationship between consumption and problem rates, typically use per capita sales figures from official sources as the explanatory variable. Average consumption per adult, 15 years or older, is often employed. On the other hand, in studies of the distribution of alcohol consumption, abstainers are commonly left out. As there may not be any strong correlation between per capita consumption per drinker and the prevalence of abstainers, the relationship between problem rates and consumption per adult may be somewhat attenuated, compared with the relationship between problem rates and consumption per drinker.

A second problem derives from the fact that unrecorded consumption is substantial in some countries. Variations in unrecorded consumption may attenuate the correlations even further.

As was noted earlier, different sociodemographic groups may sometimes change their drinking at different rates. Hence, trends in overall per capita consumption may not always be an accurate indicator of subgroup trends in problem drinking. Ideally, one would need supplementary information about group-specific changes in drinking, but these data are seldom available.

With all kinds of non-experimental data one has to face the possibility of spurious correlation: two variables may be closely correlated because they are both products of the same underlying mechanism. Basically, aggregate relationships can be studied through two different types of data. Cross-sectional comparisons can be made at any one time between different populations (ecological correlation), or time-series observations can be made on the same population at different points in time (transfer function analysis). Relationships that are based on ecological data are, for a number of technical reasons, rather ambiguous, and will not be examined in this chapter. The time-series approach can be expected to yield more reliable estimates than ecological analyses. The fundamental problem in time series is, however, the fact that two series may have coinciding trends, although they are not causally related. Similarly, phenomena that are in fact positively related may sometimes have very different trends, and may even move in opposite directions. The reason for this is typically that other relevant factors, which affect the dependent variable, are not constant over time.

The fact that most damages have a multifactorial aetiology has some important and often overlooked consequences for the interpretation of aggregate relationships between consumption and damage. The observation that a specific damage rate is stable or decreasing while consumption is increasing does not preclude the possibility of a genuine positive correlation between the two variables. The divergent trends may be the result of the ameliorating impact of causal factors other than alcohol. A study of fatal accidents in Norway provides an illustration: during the period 1951–1980 per capita consumption almost doubled in Norway whereas rates of violent deaths were quite stable (Skog 1986). Does this suggest that this form of mortality is unresponsive to changes in consumption? A closer analysis revealed that alcohol-related violent deaths had indeed increased, but this was offset by a marked decrease in industrial accidents, which are almost never alcohol induced in Norway. In this case another factor – industrial accident prevention – exerted an impact opposite to that of consumption, with the result that the alcohol effect was concealed in the overall trends. The example serves as warning against drawing incautious inferences from trend analyses.

That other factors are not 'equal' may or may not be a problem in the estimation of the effects of alcohol consumption on problem rates. Provided that modern statistical techniques are used, the situation is not problematic so long as there are no genuine correlations between consumption and other aetiological factors, which are not explicitly considered (Box and Jenkins 1976). However, if another aetiological factor is indeed related to consumption in an intimate way, then it should be brought into the model, or we risk biased estimates.

With the need for methodological caution duly underlined we will review below a number of studies on the aggregate relationship between alcohol consumption and population rates for different kinds of damage. This review is primarily based on articles published in international journals since 1979. We have chosen to put an emphasis on studies that deal satisfactorily with the methodological problems that are discussed above, while other studies, if mentioned at all, are treated more cursorily. Unfortunately, until recently, only a few methodologically adequate studies have been reported in this arena.

As was noted earlier, the relationship between consumption and damage sometimes may have a distributed time-lag structure. Whenever relevant, this has been taken into consideration in the analyses reviewed below.

4.3.2. Total mortality

Death is, manifestly, one very serious outcome which can result from drinking. In moving the discussion towards considering the relationship between population consumption and mortality rates, sight should not be lost of the fact that a large section of alcohol-related harm is social, psychological, and family related. Total mortality, the death rate, is a classical proxy for the overall health status of the population. Its association with per capita alcohol consumption is therefore of considerable interest, although the degree to which alcohol-related mortality is a satisfactory marker for the total array of health and social problems which can result from heavy drinking, requires scrutiny in any particular situation.

The findings here – based on time-series data for Prussia, France, and Sweden (Norström forthcoming) – are fairly consistent, and imply that a 1-litre increase in per capita consumption entails an increase in mortality among middle-aged men of just over 1%. Thus, a quite substantial change in per capita consumption may not leave any easily detectable trace in mortality rates. This is a reflection of the fact that drinking oneself to death is but one of several paths to eternity. It should be borne in mind, however, that even though the overall impact of consumption is hard to discern, it is certainly felt where it is concentrated; that is, in the segments of the population where heavy drinking is prevalent, and in the alcohol sector of the medical services. We should also remember that in historical terms radical shifts in per capita consumption are not uncommon (see Section 6.2), and may then bear significantly on overall mortality and ill-health.

There is no strong reason to expect the effect parameter (the size of the relationship) to be contingent upon the baseline level of consumption or the drinking culture, and there are no indications of such contingency in the data. However, the relative importance of alcohol as a risk factor – in terms of its attributable fraction as derived from the aggregate findings – is much greater in a high consumption country compared with a nation with low consumption.

4.3.3. *Specific causes of death*

If instead of total mortality, we focus on mortality where drinking is a known risk factor, the prospects for establishing the aggregate impact of consumption should be greater. This expectation is borne out in Skog's study (1987) where he analysed a more restricted category of what is usually referred to as alcohol-related mortality. This included liver cirrhosis, alcoholic psychosis, alcoholism, pancreatitis, and cancers of the upper digestive tract and of the pancreas. The temporal variation in this form of mortality was significantly related to changes in per capita consumption, and the results indicated that other factors had a restricted impact only. Thorsen (1990), in his comprehensive study based on Danish data, performed similar, but more detailed analyses (applying ARIMA models). His findings are consistent with those reported for Norway.

For other causes of death, where the aetiological significance of alcohol is only minor or less certain, the aggregate evidence is less convincing. With respect to cancer, all inclusive, it is doubtful whether any link to per capita consumption should be expected in view of the small overall aetiological importance of alcohol compared with other causes of cancer; its attributable fraction has been estimated as about 3% (Rothman 1980). Furthermore, the long period of latency, with a concomitant strong time lag, makes it even harder to discover any effects. If one instead focuses on more specific sites, where the micro evidence for a relationship with alcohol is stronger (e.g. oesophageal cancer), we encounter the problem set by a small number of deaths, in addition to the time-lag difficulty. None of what is said here should be interpreted as downplaying the significance of alcohol as a cancer risk factor at the individual level of analysis (see Section 3.6.1).

When it comes to mortality from various heart diseases, the role of alcohol is much debated, and the alleged J-shaped risk function has provoked controversy. There are, of course, echoes here of the debate which has already been explored in Chapter 3 (Section 3.5.1), in relation to individual-level data. If a J-shaped relationship pertains, the overall effects for the population should be tested by analysing the aggregate relationship. One such analysis (Skog 1983) suggested a protective impact of alcohol against ischaemic heart disease in some low-consuming population categories, although the correlation was borderline in terms of statistical significance. More extensive analyses along these lines are needed before any firm conclusions can be drawn at the population level.

4.3.4. *Cirrhosis mortality*

Mortality from cirrhosis is a classical indicator of excessive drinking (Sherlock 1982), and has received a great deal of attention in alcohol research. The risk function is firmly established in case–control studies (Pequignot *et al.* 1978), and as already mentioned, it is found to be approximately exponential. This implies that the effect on the risk of a given increase in intake depends on the level of consumption; at low levels the risk increase is small, while it is considerable at higher levels of consumption. A further implication is that the great bulk of cases will be found among the heavy drinkers. Analyses of time-series data (applying ARIMA models) for several countries, confirm previous findings of an aggregate relationship between consumption and cirrhosis based on more primitive methods (Skog 1984*a*; Norström 1987*a,b*; Thorsen 1990). In general, the response is more than proportionate, except at very low levels of consumption where the large fraction of non-alcohol related deaths makes the response less elastic. This line of research has also refined our insights about the shape of the time lag (see 4.4.1) . The findings here suggest that the total impact of a change in per capita consumption on cirrhosis mortality is distributed over an appreciable time period, in fact more than two decades. Approximately one-fifth of the impact takes place instantaneously, and within 4 years about half the effect is realized (Skog 1984*a*; Norström 1987*b*).

However, deviant case examples have indeed been reported (Grant *et al.* 1986; Smart 1988), where cirrhosis mortality has not responded as expected to changes in consumption. Several explanations seem possible. First, as was exemplified above, the marked convexity of the underlying risk function makes the aggregate association sensitive to even minor changes in the consumption distribution, particularly in its tail. Secondly, the strong time lag implies that non-uniform consumption changes across age-groups will affect the aggregate outcome.

Another confounding factor may be the introduction of mutual help organizations and large-scale treatment programmes for 'alcoholics'. Such programmes may have the effect that an appreciable number of heavy drinkers at least temporarily reduce their intake: this issue is further discussed in Chapter 9, Section 9.3.

4.3.5. *Traffic accidents*

Both experimental and epidemiological research show that driving while under the influence of alcohol entails an elevated accident risk (see Chapter 7). Since an increase in per capita consumption means more drinking occasions and larger intakes per occasion, one would expect an aggregate relationship between consumption and traffic fatalities. Although methodological and data problems mean that this expectation is not always borne out (Skog 1984*b*), several studies report positive findings. On the basis of a quasi-experimental design, utilizing US data, Cook (1981) provided evidence in the form of negative elasticities between the price of alcohol and consumption, and auto fatalities. More evidence is reported by Wagenaar (1984); an ARIMA analysis of monthly data from the state of Michigan showed a significant relationship between consumption proxies and the number of alcohol-related traffic crashes (with a 1-month lag). Thorsen (1990), on the basis of Danish data, obtained more mixed results. A time-series analysis of a change in distilled spirits availability in North Carolina, found that aggregate consumption of spirits increased, as did single vehicle night-time traffic crashes, a class of accident which is shown to have a high alcohol involvement (Blose and Holder 1987).

4.3.6. *Suicide and criminal violence*

Not until recently were social, or behavioural, alcohol-related damages, addressed in aggregate studies. Research concerning two damage rates of this kind will be included in this discussion, namely suicide and criminal violence. These two phenomena can be regarded as extreme expressions of a larger repertoire of, respectively, self-destructive and aggressive behaviours which are either unrecorded or poorly recorded, and thus not amenable to statistical analyses, but which are nevertheless likely to be influenced by drinking. Attempted suicide and domestic violence could be listed as further examples, and alcohol undoubtedly has harmful effects of this kind that reach beyond anything reflected in the mere correlations between suicide, criminal violence, and alcohol consumption.

Although the relationship is likely to be complex, it is not far-fetched to postulate some sort of causal links between alcohol and suicide. First, heavy drinking may lead to a deterioration of social ties. Secondly, the acute state of intoxication may reduce the individual's self-control and thereby trigger a suicidal inclination. Third, heavy alcohol use is associated with depression, a primary precursor of suicide. The association between heavy drinking and suicide is substantiated by a large number of epidemiological and psychiatric findings. Studies of individuals who commit suicide have repeatedly found a high incidence of 'alcoholism' (Beskow 1979). Furthermore, several follow-up studies of 'alcoholics' report grossly elevated risk-ratios for suicide (Sundby 1967; Ritson 1977). Findings of this kind may, however, be biased by selection effects which operate in such a way that the subjects who commit suicide are already at elevated risk prior to their drinking careers.

Several aggregate findings, which are not expected to carry such selection bias, do, however, suggest a link between alcohol and suicide. Two US studies have found positive relations between overall consumption and suicide rates, temporally (Wasserman 1989), as well as cross-sectionally (Rusk *et al.* 1986). On the basis of ARIMA analyses, such relations have also been confirmed for France (Norström 1988), Hungary (Skog and Elekes 1993), Norway and Sweden (Norström 1988*c*; Rossow 1993), and Denmark (Skog 1993).

A link between alcohol and violence is suggested by experimental data (Gustafson 1986), as well as by the fact that a large proportion of violent offenders are reported to have been intoxicated at the time of the crime (Mayfield 1976; Roslund and Larson 1979). The latter findings, however, do not necessarily imply a causal effect of alcohol; it is conceivable that frequent intoxication is a vital ingredient of the life-styles of violence-prone individuals. Aggregate relationships between consumption and crime rates are therefore of greater relevance for assessing the degree to which alcohol actually has an exogenous impact. Most findings here derive from Lenke's (1990) extensive study of data from France and the Nordic countries (Denmark, Finland, Norway, and Sweden). All findings are based on ARIMA analyses of fairly long time series. Statistically significant alcohol effects on assault rates are revealed for all these countries, except Denmark (the result for Norway is confirmed in a study by Skog and Björk 1988). For Sweden, the alcohol effect on the homicide rate was also significant. A series of natural experiments pertaining to Sweden provide further evidence supporting the contention that changes in per capita consumption affect violent criminality.

Considering the great cultural variation in drinking practices and drunken comportment (MacAndrew and Edgerton 1969), we might well expect national differences in the aggregate association between alcohol and social damages such as suicide and violence. Of particular interest here is the finding that the alcohol effect on suicide (Norström 1992) and criminal violence (Lenke 1990) is markedly stronger in Sweden than in France. This may be interpreted in terms of differences between dry and wet cultures with respect to drinking patterns as well as with respect to the genesis of heavy drinking, and the reaction of the environment to such behaviour.

4.3.7 *Other factors affecting aggregate problem rates*

Although the evidence which has been reviewed above supports the notion that population consumption level has an impact on the rate of alcohol problems of different kinds, it is clear that per capita consumption is not the only relevant determinant of aggregate problem rates. First, as we have already pointed out, the relationship between per capita consumption and the number of persons at risk is not mathematically exact. Second, several other dimensions, besides the long-term level of intake, are relevant in relation to many types of damage. The relevance of the general level of consumption in society will then vary across types of problems. In the case of long-term, indirect problems (for instance, social and psychological functioning), as well as direct and indirect problems of acute intoxication, it is well known that the prevalence rates do not always match the per capita consumption level closely (Mäkelä 1978).

Rates of acute alcohol problems in a society are closely linked to the way alcohol is consumed, and to cultural rules for drunken comportment. In some countries, heavy intoxication is probably more common than in other countries. Moreover, a Scandinavian with a blood–alcohol concentration of, say, 0.15 mg%, may typically behave differently from an Italian with the same blood–alcohol level. Variations of this kind should be expected to have an independent effect on rates of alcohol problems. Hence, one should not fall into the trap of supposing that since per capita consumption is so important, any measure which fails to affect per capita consumption is likely to be without effect.

In general, the relationships between per capita consumption and rates of acute alcohol problems, as well as indirect problems of long-term heavy drinking, are thus more complex than the relationship between per capita consumption and chronic disease. However, this does not imply that changes in aggregate consumption have little or no relevance to rates of acute alcohol problems. Changes in drinking patterns and the cultural rules for drunken comportment are usually quite slow. In the absence of rapid and pervasive cultural change, increasing per capita consumption will be accompanied by increasing rates of acute problems, along with increasing rates of chronic problems.

If the qualitative aspects of the drinking culture were to change, parallel with changes in per capita consumption, things might look different. For instance, if explosive drinking was gradually disappearing from the culture as the consumption level increases, one might expect increasing rates of chronic problems, and at the same time decreasing or at least stable rates of acute problems. There are hardly any historical examples of such rapid changes in drinking culture, but they are at least a theoretical possibility (Room 1992).

4.4 Aggregate drinking, alcohol-related problems, and the policy implication

Within the general structure of this book we will, as with Chapter 3, hold back from commenting piecemeal on policy implications, and at this point will do no more than signal some main conclusions. The evidence deployed in this chapter does, however, persuasively support the contention that there is today a broad base of scientific knowledge and some very firm findings on which to build rational policies.

The primary focus of the chapter has been the population rates of different types of problems. A substantial body of data demonstrate a relationship between the overall level of alcohol consumption in society and population rates of diverse types of damage, including somatic diseases resulting from long-term heavy drinking, accidents following acute intoxication, and criminal violence and suicide. Thus, the evidence supports the notion that aggregate consumption has a bearing on public health and social policy.

Nevertheless, the multiplicity of factors influencing rates of acute problems clearly indicate that an extended theoretical and policy framework, where both the quantity drunk and qualitative aspects of the drinking culture are integrated, is needed in relation to acute and more indirect problems. Hence, although overall aggregate consumption will usually have an important bearing on population health and especially on chronic health problems, it is hard to avoid the conclusion that in order to be complete, a sensible preventive strategy needs to include measures aimed both at the general level of consumption in society and at drinking patterns in a more qualitative sense – in particular, acute intoxication and cultural rules for drunken comportment, and at the contexts and social situations in which people drink. These foci for primary prevention then need to be supplemented by measures focused on particular at-risk groups. Fortunately, one does not have to choose one single item from this menu.

References

Agarwal D. and Goedde H. (1991) The role of alcohol metabolising enzymes in alcohol sensitivity, alcohol drinking habits, and the incidence of alcoholism in orientals. In Palmer N.T. (ed.) *The Molecular Pathology of Alcoholism*, pp. 211–237. Oxford University Press.

Aitchison J. and Brown J.A.C. (1969) *The Lognormal Distribution*. Cambridge: Cambridge University Press.

Anastasi A. (1958) *Differential Psychology and Group Differences in Behaviour*. New York: Macmillan.

Ball D.M. and Murray R.M. (1994) Genetics of alcohol misuse. In: Edwards

G. and Peters T.J. (eds.) *Alcohol Misuse. British Medical Bulletin* Vol. 50, pp. 18–35..

Beskow J. (1979). Suicide and mental disorder in Swedish men. *Acta Psychiatrica Scandinavica, Supplementum* 277.

Blinder A.S. (1974) *Towards an Economic Theory of Income Distribution.* Cambridge, MA: MIT Press.

Blose J. and Holder H.D. (1987). Liquor-by-the-drink and alcohol-related traffic crashes: A natural experiment using time-series analysis. *Journal of Studies on Alcohol* **48**, 52–60.

Box G.E.P. and Jenkins G.M. (1976). *Time Series Analysis: Forecasting and Control.* London: Holdens-Day, Inc.

Bruun K., Edwards G., Lumio M., Mälelä K., Pan L., Popham R.E., *et al.* 1975. *Alcohol Control Policies in Public Health Perspective.* Helsinki: The Finnish Foundation for Alcohol Studies.

Clark W.R. and Hilton M.E. (1991) *Alcohol in America: Drinking Practices and Problems.* Albany, NY: State University of New York Press.

Cook C.C.H. and Gurling H.M.D. (1991) Genetic factors in alcoholism. In: Palmer N.T. (ed.) *The Molecular Pathology of Alcoholism*, pp. 182–210. Oxford University Press.

Cook P.J. (1981) The effect of liquor taxes on drinking, cirrhosis, and auto accidents. In: Moore M.H. and Gerstein D.R. (eds.) *Alcohol and Public Policy: Beyond the Shadow of Prohibition*, pp. 255–258. Washington, DC: National Academy Press.

Duffy J. (1986) The distribution of alcohol consumption: 30 years on. *British Journal of Addiction* **73**, 259–264.

Edwards G., Gross M.M., Keller M., Moser J., and Room R. (1977) *Alcohol-related Disabilities.* Geneva: World Health Organization.

Grant B., Noble J., and Malin H. (1986) Decline in liver cirrhosis mortality and components of change: United States, 1973–1983. *Alcohol Health and Research World*, **10**, 66–69.

Gustafson R. (1986) *Alcohol and human physical aggression: the mediating role of frustration.* Department of Psychology, University of Uppsala (Dissertation).

Jaffe J.H. (1988) Some differential effects of genes and environment on alcoholism. In: Rose R.M. and Barrett J.E. (ed.) *Alcoholism: Origins and Outcome*, pp. 75–82. New York: Raven Press.

Jolliffe N. and Jellinek E.M. (1941). Vitamin deficiencies and liver cirrhosis in alcoholism. Part VII. Cirrhosis of the liver. *Quarterly Journal of Studies on Alcohol* **2**, 544–583.

Kendell R.E. (1987) Drinking sensibly. *British Journal of Addiction* **82**, 1279–1288.

Kreitman N. (1986) Alcohol consumption and the preventive paradox. *British Journal of Addiction* **81**, 353–363.

Ledermann S. (1956) *Alcool, Alcoolism, Alcoolisation*, Vol. I. Paris: Presses Universitaires de France.

Ledermann S. (1964) *Alcool, Alcoolism, Alcoolisation*, Vol. 2. Paris: Presses Universitaires de France.

Lemmens P., Tan E., and Knibbe R. (1990) Comparing distributions of alcohol consumption: empirical probability plots. *British Journal of Addiction* **85**, 751–58.

Lenke L. (1990). *Alcohol and Criminal Violence – Time Series Analyses in a Comparative Perspective*. Stockholm: Almqvist and Wiksell.

MacAndrew C. and Edgerton R.B. (1969). *Drunken Comportment*. Chicago: Aldine.

Mäkelä K. (1969). *Alkoholinkulutuksen jakautuma*. (Mimeo). Helsinki: Social Research Institute for Alcohol Studies.

Mäkelä K. (1978) Levels of consumption and social consequences of drinking, In: Israel, Y., Glaser F.B., Kalant H., Popham R.E., Schmidt W., and Smart R.C. (ed.) *Research Advances in Alcohol and Drug Problems*, pp. 303–349. New York: Plenum Press.

Mäkelä K., Room R., Single E., Sulhunen P., and Walsh B. (1981) *Alcohol, Society and the State*. Toronto: Addiction Research Foundation.

Mayfield D. (1976) Alcoholism, alcohol, intoxication and assaultative behavior. *Diseases of the Nervous System* **37**, 288–291.

Moore M.H. and Gerstein D.R. (1981) *Alcohol and Public Policy: Beyond the Shadow of Prohibition*. Washington, DC: National Academy Press.

Norström T. (1987*a*). The abolition of the Swedish alcohol rationing system: Effects on consumption distribution and cirrhosis mortality. *British Journal of Addiction* **82**, 633–642.

Norström T. (1987*b*) The impact of per capita consumption on Swedish cirrhosis mortality. *British Journal of Addiction* **82**, 67–75.

Norström T. (1988). Alcohol and suicide in Scandinavia. *British Journal of Addiction* **83**, 553–559.

Norström T. (forthcoming) Alcohol and damages: the aggregate evidence.

Nutt D. (1994) The changing pharmacology of addiction. In: Edwards G. and Lader M. (ed.) *Addiction: Processes of Change*, pp. 33–49. Oxford University Press.

Partanen J., Bruun K., and Markkanen T. (1966) *Inheritance of Drinking Behavior*. Helsinki: Finnish Foundation for Alcohol Studies.

Pequignot G., Tuyns A., and Bertha J.L. (1978) Ascitic cirrhosis in relation to alcohol consumption. *International Journal of Epidemiology* **7**, 113–120.

Popham R.E. (1970) Indirect methods of alcoholism prevalence estimation: A critical evaluation. In: Popham R.E. (ed.) *Alcohol and Alcoholism*, pp. 294–306. University of Toronto Press.

Popham R.E. and Schmidt W. (1976). Some factors affecting the likelihood of moderate drinking by treated alcoholics. *Journal of Studies on Alcohol* **37**, 868–882.

Ritson B. (1977). Alcoholism and suicide. In: Edwards G. and Grant M. (ed.) *Alcoholism. New Knowledge and New Responses*, pp. 271–8. London: Croom Helm.

Room R. (1992) The impossible dream? Routes to reducing alcohol problems in a temperance culture. *Journal of Substance Abuse* **4**, 91–106.

Rose G. (1981) Strategy of prevention: lessons from cardiovascular diseases. *British Medical Journal* **282**, 1847–1851.

Roslund B. and Larson C.A. (1979) Crimes of violence and alcohol abuse in Sweden. *The International Journal of the Addictions* **14**, 1103–1115.

Rossow I. (1993) Suicide, alcohol, and divorce: aspects of gender and family integration. *Addiction* **88**, 1659–1665.

Rothman K.J. (1980) The proportion of cancer attributable to alcohol consumption. *Preventive Medicine* **9**, 174–179.

Rusk B., Gliksman L., and Brook R. (1986). Alcohol availability, alcohol consumption and alcohol-related damage. I. The distribution of consumption model. *Journal of Studies on Alcohol* **47**, 1–10.

Sherlock S. (ed.) 1982. *Alcohol and Disease*. London: Churchill Livingstone.

Simpura J. (1985). *Alcohol Consumption and the Shape of its Distribution by Sex and Age in Four Scandinavian Countries*. Paper presented at the ICAA Alcohol Epidemiology Section, Rome, June 1985.

Skog O.-J. (1979). *Modeller for drikkeatferd (Models of Drinking Behaviour)*. SIFA-report No. 32. Oslo: National Institute for Alcohol Research.

Skog O.-J. (1980*a*) Social interaction and the distribution of alcohol consumption. *Journal of Drug Issues* **10**, 71–92.

Skog O.-J. (1980*b*) Liver cirrhosis epidemiology: Some methodological problems. *British Journal of Addiction* **75**, 227–243.

Skog O.-J. (1983) Methodological problems in the analysis of temporal covariation between alcohol consumption and ischemic heart disease. *British Journal of Addiction* **78**, 157–172.

Skog O.-J. (1984*a*) The risk function for liver cirrhosis from lifetime alcohol consumption. *Journal of Studies on Alcohol* **45**, 199–208.

Skog O.-J. (1984*b*) *Ökt totalforbruk – flere trafikkulykker?* (Higher per capita consumption – more traffic accidents?) SIFA-Report No. 87/84. Oslo: National Institute for Alcohol Research.

Skog O.-J. (1985*a*) Hva bestemmer omfanget av alkoholskader? (What determines the aggregate volume of alcohol problems?) In: Arner O., Hauge R., and Skog O.-J. (ed.) *Alkohol i Norge*, pp. 190–211. Oslo: Universitetsforlaget.

Skog O.-J. (1985*b*) The wetness of drinking cultures: A key variable in epidemiology of alcoholic liver cirrhosis. *Acta Medica Scandinavica* Suppl. 703, 157–184.

Skog O.-J. (1985*c*) The collectivity of drinking cultures. A theory of the distribution of alcohol consumption. *British Journal of Addiction* **80**, 83–99.

Skog O.-J. (1986) Trends in alcohol consumption and violent deaths. *British Journal of Addiction* **81**, 365–379.

Skog O.-J. (1987) Trends in alcohol consumption and deaths from diseases. *British Journal of Addiction* **82**, 1033–1041.

Skog O.-J. (1991) Drinking and the distribution of alcohol consumption. In: Pittman D.J. and White H.R. (ed.) *Society, Culture and Drinking Patterns Reexamined*, pp. 135–156. New Brunswick, NJ: Rutgers Center of Alcohol Studies.

Skog O.-J. (1992) Epidemiological and biostatistical aspects of alcohol use, alcoholism, and their complications. In: Erickson P.G. and Kalant, H. (ed.) *Windows on Science*, pp. 3–35. Toronto: Addiction Research Foundation.

Skog O.-J. (1993). Alcohol and suicide in Denmark 1911–24 – experiences from a 'natural experiment'. *Addiction* **88**, 1189–1193.

Skog O.-J. and Björk E. (1988). Alkohol og voldskriminalitet: En analyse av utviklingen i Norge 1931–1982 (Alcohol and crimes of violence: an analysis of the development in Norway 1931–1982). *Nordisk Tidskrift for Kriminalvidenskab* **75**, 1–23.

Skog O.-J. and Duckert F. (1993). The development of alcoholics' and heavy drinkers' consumption: A longitudinal study. *Journal of Studies on Alcohol* **54**, 178–188.

Skog O.-J. and Elekes S. (1993). Alcohol and the 1950–90 Hungarian suicide trend – is there a causal connection? *Acta Sociologica* **36**, 33–46.

Smart R.G. (1988) Recent international reductions and increases in liver cirrhosis deaths. *Alcoholism. Clinical and Experimental Research* **12**, 239–242.

Sundby P. (1967) *Alcoholism and Mortality*. Stockholm: Almqvist and Wiksell.

Thorsen T. (1990). *Hundrede ars alkoholmisbrug*. Copenhagen: Alkohol- og Narkotikartådet.

Vaillant G.E. (1988) Some differential effects of genes and environment on alcoholism. In: Rose R.M. and Barrett J.E. (ed.) *Alcoholism: Origins and Outcome*. pp. 75–82. New York: Raven Press.

Wagenaar A.C. (1984) Alcohol consumption and the incidence of acute alcohol-related problems. *British Journal of Addiction* **79**, 173–180.

Wasserman I. M. (1989) The effects of war and alcohol consumption patterns on suicide: United States, 1910–1933. *Social Forces* **68**, 513–530.

Part II

Multiple policy options and the
evidence for their efficacy

5

Retail price influences on alcohol consumption, and taxation of alcohol as a prevention strategy

There are many determinants of drinking besides the cost factor. The micro-environment, social learning and the collectivity of the 'drinking culture' (pp. 90–1), constitution as defined in both psychological and physical terms (pp. 92–4), and the whole range of social and cultural influences that may impact on national consumption are some of the factors which must be taken into consideration. Price must be discussed within this total context.

But within that context one must take note of the fact that humans are economic animals. That aphorism might be seen as finding support in the unpopularity of the budget which puts a penny on the pint of beer, the ready trade in bottles conducted by the duty-free airport shop, the popularity of the happy hour, or the Skid Row alcoholic's sad resort to methylated spirits or rubbing alcohol. Lay wisdom would thus suggest that the price of alcohol is likely to bear tangibly on its consumption.

The reason for writing a chapter on this topic lies in the belief that within the total flow of interactive influences, the cost of beverage alcohol is one potent influence bearing on the level and occasions of its consumption. Price is not the only factor determining how the individual and the population imbibe, but price will interact with every other kind of informal and formal control. Taxation is thus a potential instrument to be used in the health interest.

The structure of this chapter will be as follows. In Section 5.1 the relevant econometric concepts will be outlined. This will be followed in 5.2 and under a general 'research evidence' heading, by discussion of findings relating in sequence to the price elasticity of alcohol, and situations which may influence these elasticities; the substitution problem; evidence relating to the impact of dramatic price change; the differential impact of price on different sections of the population, and in particular the question of whether price is likely to influence the drinking of 'the addict'. These background considerations lead up to Section 5.3, and discussion of the likely efficacy of taxation as a public health measure.

5.1 Price elasticity as an economic concept

The sensitivity of demand to price change is called *price elasticity*, defined as the unit change in demand caused by a unit change in price. This is usually expressed as percentage change. For instance, the price elasticity of beer is the per cent change in demand for beer – increase or decrease – in direct response to a 1% change in the price of beer to the consumer. In like manner, income as one indicator of the economic ability of the consumer to purchase a commodity, has its own elasticity with reference to alcohol, and this is called *income elasticity*. Elasticities for other supply factors can also be estimated. For instance the sensitivity of consumption to changes in the number of liquor stores has been estimated in many studies (see p. 134), as well as an elasticity measuring the effects of changes in alcohol advertising.

A product can be described as *price elastic, price inelastic*, or as having a *unit price elasticity*. That a product is price elastic means that the per cent change in quantity demanded is greater than the operative per cent change in the price of the product. Similarly, a product being price inelastic indicates that the per cent change in quantity demanded is smaller than the change in price of the product; that a product is price inelastic does not therefore imply that it will show no response to a price change, but only that the change in demand in response to a 1% increase is less than 1%, and thus less than for a product which is price elastic. Unit price elasticity means that the per cent change in quantity demanded is exactly the same as the per cent change in the product price.

Some studies include lag terms to account for long-term adjustments in demand. The short-run price elasticity gives the immediate effect, and the long-term price elasticity the total effect of change in price on consumption.

5.2 Alcohol consumption and price: the research evidence

The effect of price change on alcohol consumption has been more extensively investigated than any other potential alcohol policy measure. Most commonly these investigations have relied on econometric methods but they also include panel studies, observational studies, and analysis of major changes in alcohol prices. There are econometric studies dealing with total consumption or discreet beverage categories, and relevant research is available from at least the following countries: Australia, Belgium, Canada, Denmark, Germany, Finland, France, Ireland, Italy, Kenya, the Netherlands, New Zealand, Norway, Portugal, Spain, Sweden, the

United Kingdom, and the USA (Bruun *et al.* 1975; Ornstein and Levy 1983; Godfrey 1986; Clements and Selvanathan 1991; Partanen 1991). Knowledge of the effects of alcohol prices on alcohol consumption mainly comes from Western industrial countries.

The values of price elasticities for alcohol have consistently shown that when other factors remain unchanged, a rise in price has generally led to a drop in consumption. Similarly, a decrease in price has usually led to a rise in consumption. In the same manner, income elasticities estimated in different studies have shown that when other factors remain unchanged, a rise in consumer disposable income has generally led to consumption going up while a decrease has led to a depression in demand.

Alcohol appears, therefore, as with other commodities, to be subject to economic laws of supply and demand. The demand for the product is responsive to the actual retail cost to the consumer. In general, as a product becomes more costly relative to other goods and services, demand for it is reduced, and as a product becomes in those terms less costly, demand is increased.

5.2.1 *Values of price elasticities*

Table 5.1 summarizes a set of econometric studies by country. The time period is also shown. Almost all price elasticity values have an absolute value greater than zero and are negative, indicating that changes in price affect consumption in a direction consistent with economic theory. Put simply, there is a robust finding that if prices go up consumption goes down, and if prices go down consumption goes up. However, the actual values of price elasticities for different beverages and for different countries and over time, are not uniform.

To look a little more closely at the detailed implications of this core finding, if the demand for a given category of beverage is price elastic (relatively sensitive to price change), a rise in price will have a relatively strong diminishing effect on consumption, and decrease the share of personal disposable income allocated to that beverage. Similarly, a decline in price will have a relatively strong positive effect on consumption, and increase the share of personal disposable income allocated to that beverage. In Table 5.1 this scenario is illustrated with spirits in Canada in 1949–1969, wine in Norway in 1960–1974, and with strong beer in Sweden in 1956–1968.

In the same manner, if the demand for a given category of beverage is price inelastic (relatively insensitive to price change), a rise in price will cause a relatively small diminution in demand, and will increase the share of personal disposable income allocated to that beverage. A decline in price will have a relatively slight positive effect on consumption and decrease the

Table 5.1. Price elasticities of beer, wine, and distilled spirits

Author	Place	Time	Beer	Wine	Distilled spirits
Lau (1975)	Canada	1949–1969	−0.03	−1.65	−1.45
Johnson and Oksanen (1974)	Canada	1955–1971[1]	−0.22	−0.50	−0.91
	Canada	1955–1971[2]	−0.38	−1.30	−1.60
Johnson and Oksanen (1977)	Canada	1955–1971[1]	−0.27	−0.67	−1.14
	Canada	1955–71	−0.33	−1.78	−1.77
Quek (1988)	Canada	1953–1982	−0.28	−0.58	−0.30
Johnson et al. (1992)	Canada	1956–1983[1]	−0.26 to −0.31	−0.70 to −0.88	−0.45 to −0.82
		1956–1983[2]	−0.14	−1.17	NA
Niskanen (1962)	USA	1934–1960	−0.50	−1.59	−2.03
	USA	1934–1960	−0.33	−0.35	−0.93
Hogarty and Elzinga (1972)	USA	1956–1959	−0.89	NA	NA
Simon (1966)	USA	1955–1961	NA	NA	−0.79
Comanor & Wilson (1974)	USA	1947–1964[1]	−0.56	−0.68	−0.25
	USA	1947–1964[2]	−1.39	−0.84	−0.30
Norman (1975)	USA	1946–1970	−0.87	NA	NA
Smith (1976)	USA	1970	NA	NA	−1.95
Labys (1976)	USA	1954–1971	NA	−0.44[5]/−1.65[6]	NA
Lidman (1976)	California	1953–1975	NA	NA	0.02
Clements and Selvanathan (1987)	USA	1949–1982	−0.09	−0.22	−0.10
Selvanathan (1991)	USA	1949–1982	−0.11	−0.05	−0.11
Eecen (1985)	Netherlands	1960–1983	0.0	−0.5	NA
Labys (1976)/EEC (1972)	Belgium	1954–1971	NA	−1.14	NA
Labys (1976)	France	1954–1971	NA	−0.06	NA
Labys (1976)	Italy	1954–1971	NA	−1.00	NA
Labys (1976)	Portugal	1954–1971	NA	−0.68	NA
Labys (1976)	Spain	1954–1971	NA	−0.37	NA

TABLE 4.1 cont.

Author	Place	Time	Beer	Wine	Distilled spirits
Labys (1976)	Germany (Fed. Rep.)	1954–1971	NA	−0.38	NA
Walsh and Walsh (1970)	Ireland	1953–1967	−0.17	NA	−0.64
Prest (1949)	United Kingdom	1870–1938	−0.66	NA	−0.57
Wong (1988)	United Kingdom	1920–1938	−0.25	−0.99	−0.51
Stone (1945)	United Kingdom	1920–1938	−0.73	NA	−0.72
Stone (1951)	United Kingdom	1920–1948	−0.69	−1.17[6]	−0.57
Walsh (1982)	United Kingdom	1955–1975	−0.13	−0.28	−0.47
Clements and Selvanathan (1987)	United Kingdom	1955–1975	−0.19	−0.23	−0.24
McGuinness (1983)	United Kingdom	1956–1979	−0.30	−0.17	−0.38
Duffy (1983)	United Kingdom	1963–1978	NA	−1.0	−0.77
Godfrey (1988)	United Kingdom	1956–1980	NA	−0.76 to −1.14	−0.88 to −0.98
		1956–1980	NA	−0.91	−0.56 to −0.99
Duffy (1987)	United Kingdom	1963–1983	−0.29	−0.77	−0.51
Selvanathan (1988)	United Kingdom	1955–1985	−0.13	−0.37	−0.32
Jones (1989)	United Kingdom	1964–1983	−0.27	−0.77	−0.95
			−0.40	−0.94	−0.79
Selvanathan (1991)	United Kingdom	1955–1985	−0.13	−0.40	−0.31
Baker and McKay (1990)	United Kingdom	1970–1986	−0.88	−1.37	−0.94
Duffy (1991)	United Kingdom	1963–1983	−0.09	−0.75	−0.86
Nyberg (1967)	Finland	1949–1962	−0.49	−0.83	−0.13[3]/−0.95[4]
		1949–1962[1]	0.00	−0.99	−0.60[3]/−1.10[4]
		1949–1962[2]	+0.01	−3.28	−2.00[3]/−3.65[4]
Salo (1990)	Finland	1969–1986	−0.6	−1.3	−1.0
Horverak (1979)	Norway	1960–1974	NA	−1.5	−1.2
Malmqvist (1948)	Sweden	1923–1939	NA	−0.9	−0.3

Table 5.1 *cont.*

Author	Place	Time	Beer	Wine	Distilled spirits
Bryding and Rosén (1969)	Sweden	1920–1951	−1.2	−1.6	−0.5
Sundström-Ekström (1962)	Sweden	1931–1954	NA	−1.6	−0.3
Huitfeldt and Jorner (1972)	Sweden	1956–1968	−3.0[7]	−0.7	−1.2
Miller and Roberts (1972)	Australia	1957–1971	NA	−1.8	NA
Clements and Selvanathan (1987)	Australia	1956–1977	−0.12	−0.34	−0.52
Clements and Johnson (1983)	Australia	1956–1977	−0.11	−0.40	−0.53
Selvanathan (1991)	Australia	1955–1985	−0.15	−0.60	−0.61
Clements and Selvanathan (1991)	Australia	1956–1986	−0.15	−0.32	−0.61
Pearce (1986)	New Zealand	1966–1982	−0.15	−0.35	−0.32
Wette *et al* (1993)	New Zealand	1983–1991	−1.1	−1.1	−0.5
Partanen (1991)	Kenya	1963–1985[1]	−0.33	NA	NA
		1963–1985[2]	−1.00	NA	NA

[1] Short run.
[2] Long run.
[3] Vodka.
[4] Other spirits.
[5] Domestic.
[6] Imported.
[7] Strong beer.

share of personal disposable income allocated to that beverage. According to Table 5.1 this happened in relation to wine drinking in France during 1954–1971, beer in Ireland in 1953–1967, and spirits in Australia over the period 1956–1977.

Finally, if the demand for a given category of beverage is unit price elastic, a rise in price will have a diminishing effect on consumption of equal proportion and keep the share of personal disposable income allocated to that beverage about equal. In the obverse case a fall in price will have a positive effect on consumption of equal proportion and keep the share of personal disposable income allocated to that beverage about level. This was approximately the case with distilled spirits in Finland during 1969–1986, with wine in Italy for 1954–1971, as well as for beer in Kenya 1963–1985.

The impact of changes in price on revenue income will depend both on the elasticity values and on which components of the price are causing the change. If the change is due to production and distribution costs, the impact on government revenue will be proportional to the impact on consumption. The situation is more complex when the price change is due to taxation. In many but not all situations, a tax rise will increase government revenue even when the demand is price elastic and total expenditure on alcohol goes down. To take an extreme example, raising a levy on a previously untaxed beverage will swell revenue even if the beverage is highly price elastic, and the higher price level causes a large reduction in consumption. Only in situations where the tax rate already is high are added taxes likely to cut revenue when consumption goes down.

When talking about relatively small or large price effects on alcohol consumption, one is referring to a unit change in price. Hence, even in circumstances where the demand is price inelastic, a big absolute change in price will have a larger effect on consumption than only a slight change in price in a situation where alcohol demand is price elastic. Degree of price change as well as the value of the relevant elasticity must therefore jointly be taken into the reckoning when predicting the impact of price on consumption. We will look at the 'dramatic changes' question in 5.2.4 below.

The impact of changes in price over time may be stronger than their immediate effects (Ornstein and Levy 1983). Studies in Canada (Johnson and Oksanen 1977), the USA (Comanor and Wilson 1974), and Kenya (Partanen 1991), indicate that the short-term price elasticity has a smaller absolute value than a long-term price elasticity.

5.2.2 *Situations which may be associated with variation in the price elasticity*

The discussion above has demonstrated the utility of price elasticity as a construct describing the relationship between price change on the one hand, and change in consumption on the other. But as already emphasized the data also indicate that elasticity values are not universals. The observed variations are in part due to modelling techniques and the quality of the data. The disparities also stem from differing social, cultural, and economic circumstances prevailing in different regions and over different periods.

In English-speaking countries, it has been a common finding that the demand for beer has been less price elastic than the demand for wines and spirits. In their detailed evaluation of 20 studies, Ornstein and Levy (1983) concluded that the best estimates of price elasticities for beer, wine, and distilled spirits in the USA (and Canada) are −0.3, −1.0, and −1.5 respectively. In her discussion of several recent drink demand studies in the United Kingdom, Godfrey (1989, 1990) similarly showed that the demand for beer in the United Kingdom has generally been price inelastic. On the other hand, demand for wines and spirits has been more price responsive. In contrast to this, there are studies to indicate that the demand for wines can be relatively unresponsive to price in France and Spain (Table 5.1).

One further way to understand the basis of these disparities is to consider the different uses to which alcoholic beverages are put. Here one has to take into account the many different culturally embedded meanings given to an alcoholic drink, for instance, as an intoxicant, a thirst quencher, an accompaniment to meals, a medicine, or a means of recreation and enjoyment. Within that perspective it is no wonder that the demand for alcoholic beverages can respond very differently to a given price change in different countries and cultures, and across different periods. The interpretation of elasticity values therefore calls for an informed understanding of drinking habits in the specific society and at a point in time.

Elasticity values may further vary depending on the price level of alcoholic drinks. Under some circumstances, the value of the price elasticity may decrease as prices go down, and increase as prices go up. There was a sharp increase in liquor prices in Sweden after the repeal in 1955 of the rationing system for purchase of distilled spirits. As a consequence, there was a rise in the absolute value of the price elasticity for distilled beverages (Huifeldt and Jorner 1972). A contributing factor may have been that rationing curbed the influence of price changes on consumption. The Swedish example thus illustrates the interaction between prices and legal restriction on the availability of alcohol.

Elasticity values may also change as a consequence of increasing affluence, and of changes in the social and cultural position of alcoholic beverages. In Finland, the absolute value of the price elasticity for total alcohol consumption decreased steadily between 1955 and 1980 from −0.93

to −0.70 (Ahtola *et al.* 1986). Over that period, rising affluence and more relaxed control greatly increased the availability of alcohol. As alcohol consumption grew from under 2 litres per capita from the mid-1950s to about 6.5 litres by the early 1980s, the value of the price elasticity tended to decrease as alcohol came more and more to be used as an everyday commodity.

5.2.3 *The economics of substitution*

Because all alcoholic beverages include ethanol, they can be expected potentially to substitute for each other. But it is also evident that alcoholic beverages can serve as substitutes for, and can be replaced by, other commodities. This implies that the level of alcohol consumption, and the way in which it is consumed, can be influenced by the price of these beverages relative to other commodities.

If the price of one category of beverage is increased, then consumers may seek other less expensive licit alternatives. For example, if spirit prices are put up, the demand for wine, or beer, or both, may increase. A number of studies have developed estimates of *cross-price elasticity* – that is, of the change in demand for one category of alcoholic beverage caused by a change in the price of some other category of alcoholic beverage (Niskanen 1962; Nyberg 1967; Walsh and Walsh 1970; Huitfeldt and Jorner 1972; Johnson and Oksanen 1974; Lau 1975; Lidman 1976; Johnson and Oksanen 1977; Ornstein 1980; Godfrey 1986). The estimation of cross-elasticities has proved to be an extremely difficult task. The substitution of one type of beverage for another has, however, usually been found to be only within a modest range, with cross-price elasticities small or insignificant.

Like own price elasticities, the cross-price elasticities between different categories of alcohol are not inherent attributes of alcoholic beverages but reflections of the prevailing drinking habits and culture. In a culture where spirits and beer are drunk at the same sitting, a rise in the price of spirits may, for instance, decrease the consumption of both. Although substitution is often found to occur, it would be unwise to assume that alcoholic beverages will always substitute for each other.

In some studies it has also been observed that heavy consumers prefer the cheaper product within each type of alcoholic beverage. In such circumstances, the substitution between different types is not so much determined by changes in the average price of each category of beverage as by changes in the price of the cheapest brands in each category. Similarly, the relative price of alcohol in different categories affects which categories will behave as substitutes. It is possible that an increase in spirit prices would, for example, shift consumption from spirits to beer in some countries, to wine in other countries, or even have different consequences in the same country at a different period.

All studies of price elasticities have been based on recorded sales of alcohol and do not take into account unrecorded sources of consumption such as home production or smuggling. In designing alcohol tax policies, their potential effect on those types of consumption should be carefully monitored.

The substitution of other goods as replacement for alcohol may lead either to healthier or unhealthier habits. A rise in the price of wine, for instance, may result in substitution by soft drinks, a switch to home-produced wine, or to dangerous illicit alcohol. Substitution can be affected by controls aimed at those substances to which consumers are apt to move. If prices of legally produced alcohol are, however, kept constant or lowered because of worry over a potential substitution by illicit alcohol, the harmful effects of the legitimate alcohol may exceed the feared dangers arising from contaminated alcohol.

5.2.4 *Swinging taxes: the impact of dramatic price changes on alcohol consumption*

Econometric studies for the most part use as their material changes in alcohol prices which are small. A classic example of dramatic change comes from Denmark. Due to the food shortage during the First World War, the price of Danish aquavit was raised more than 10 times over, while the price of beer was doubled. These drastic measures reduced the per capita consumption of alcohol by three-quarters, from 6.7 to 1.6 litres, within 2 years. Not only was the total consumption affected, but the recorded cases of delirium tremens declined to one-thirteenth, and deaths due to 'alcoholismus chronicus' to one-sixth of the previous level (Bruun *et al.* 1975).

Other available examples of steep price changes are not on that kind of scale, but have taken place more recently. For instance, in Sweden, in 1957 and 1958 the real price of potable spirits went up by more than 30%. This contributed to a decline in spirit consumption from not quite 0.8 litres per capita per month in 1956, to 0.6 litres in 1958, a decrease of one-quarter (Huitfeldt and Jorner 1972).

5.2.5 *Are heavier or dependent drinkers likely to be affected by price change?*

In econometric studies based on time series, the values of price elasticities reflect the average reaction of the population to changes in price. Although it can be inferred that a rise in price will reduce consumption, that kind of research cannot by itself determine who are the people that cut down on their consumption and by how much. How is the cut distributed? Few studies address directly the differential effects of price on various groups of consumers. The evidence available, however, strongly indicates that heavy and dependent drinkers are at least as responsive to price as are more moderate consumers.

Grossman *et al.* (1987) and Coate and Grossman (1988) have in the USA studied the price sensitivity of alcohol for young people who are drinking. They found evidence that heavy drinkers are more sensitive to price changes than moderate drinkers. Kendell *et al.* (1983) studied the effect of price on consumption in Scotland with two surveys, the second being conducted after a rise in price of alcohol. The design of the study does not warrant absolutely confident conclusions (Altman 1991), but the impact of the price increase seems to have been strongest among the heaviest drinkers, both men and women. Heavy drinkers also experienced the largest reduction in the number of adverse effects related to alcohol consumption.

'Happy hours' (periods of price reduction in a pub, bar, or restaurant, or by analogy in an experimental condition), offer a possibility for studying directly the effect of decreasing prices on consumption of heavy drinkers. A study by Babor *et al.* (1978) observed heavy and light male drinkers in a hospital setting. Their patterns of drinking were examined under happy hour or non-happy hour experimental conditions. As expected both light and heavy drinkers drank more when drinks were less expensive. Light drinkers in the experimental setting drank about twice as much, and heavy drinkers drank about 2.4 times as much as when in the non-happy hour condition.

Perhaps the strongest evidence for an impact of prices on heavy and dependent drinkers comes from economic studies examining the relationship between alcohol prices and alcohol problems, particularly cirrhosis of the liver. Cirrhosis mortality is a well established indicator for the prevalence of heavy drinking. Cook adopted Simon's (1966) approach, using as a quasi-experiment the changes in state liquor excise-tax rates legislated between 1960 and 1975 in American states. Cook (1981) discovered that the states that raised their liquor tax had a greater reduction or smaller increase in cirrhosis mortality than others in the corresponding year. A follow-up study by Cook and Tauchen (1982) estimated the median price elasticity for liquor to be -1.8, and showed that liquor consumption, including that of heavy drinkers (as indicated by cirrhosis mortality), was responsive to price, with liquor tax increases also tending to reduce traffic crash fatality rates. They concluded that an increase in a state's alcohol excise tax lowers death rates by a larger percentage than it lowers per capita alcohol consumption.

5.3 Taxation as a public health strategy

The research findings reviewed in this chapter substantiate the contention that the drinker is, like a citizen who purchases any other commodity, likely to be responsive to price. Furthermore, the heavy drinker who is imperilling his or her health, is no exception to this rule.

If price influences consumption, it is not surprising on the basis of the relationship between consumption and problems discussed at individual level (Chapter 3), and population level (Chapter 4), that price should be found to bear on problem occurrence. The findings suggest the need for a subtle and contextually sensitive approach to analysis of the health benefits which may derive from use of pricing as a public health instrument. The sensibly moderate conclusion must be that taxation is likely to be useful in support of, and alliance with, other public health measures directed at curtailing the health and social burden resulting from drinking.

Four objections to the use of alcohol taxation as a public health instrument are sometimes heard. First, and particularly in a developing country, a price increase imposed on commercial beverages may stimulate illicit or home production. That danger should be heeded and monitored, but as already noted, letting commercial production go unfettered because of this fear carries its own risks (p. 118). Secondly, the budgetary authorities may view the tax obtained from beverage alcohol as a valuable and easily collectable revenue, and be reluctant to impose tax increases for fear of a consequent net loss in takings. Only a knowledge of the elasticities which are pertaining in particular circumstances can answer that question (p. 115), but in most situations a price increase will swell rather than depress the tax take. The third objection to taxation as a control measure is that such an approach is not socially equitable, with tax increases imposing a proportionally greater burden on the poorer segment of the population. The evidence available from New Zealand, the United Kingdom, and the USA does not, however, support this contention, since alcohol taxes will in most circumstances impose a lower relative burden on low-income groups than most other commodity taxes (Harris 1984; Ashton *et al.* 1989) The fourth point to be considered is that the efficacy of fiscal control may in some circumstances be eroded where borders are long or open. That speaks to the need for a strong voice to be given to health advocacy at the international level when trade and customs deals are being struck.

The impact of taxation on alcohol consumption should be viewed as an intervention in a complex system, and in that kind of situation to ignore the significance of the various provisos which have been identified would be unwise. Economic influences, we have argued, do not operate in a vacuum. At the same time the research conclusively demonstrates that the contention which is sometimes heard that taxation is irrelevant to public health, is factually unsustainable. The reasonable middle ground conclusion to be drawn from the bulk of the evidence can be stated in the following summary terms. Other things being equal, a population's consumption of alcohol will in lesser or greater but usually significant degree, be influenced by price. Heavier drinkers as well as lighter drinkers will be thus responsive, and the connection between price and consumption is likely to have its follow-through in a connection between price and population level experience of problems. And it is those linked facts that finally lead in on to the conclusion that taxation is a potentially useful lever for public health.

References

Altman D.G. (1991) *Practical Statistics for Medical Research*. London: Chapman & Hall.

Ashton T., Casswell S., and Gilmore L. (1989) Alcohol taxes: do the poor pay more than the rich? *British Journal of Addiction* **84**, 759–766.

Babor T.F., Mendelson H., Greenberg I., and Kuehnle J. (1978) Experimental analysis of the 'happy hour': effects of purchase price on alcohol consumption. *Psychopharmacology* **58**, 34–41.

Baker P. and McKay S. (1990) *The Structure of Alcohol Taxes: A Hangover from the Past?* London: The Institute for Fiscal Studies.

Bruun K., Edwards G., Lumio M., Mäkelä M., Pan L., Popham R.E., *et al.* 1975 *Alcohol Control Policies in Public Health Perspective*, Vol. 25. Helsinki: The Finnish Foundation for Alcohol Studies.

Bryding G. and Rosén U. (1969) Konsumtionen av alkoholhaltiga drycker 1920–1951, en efterfrågeanalytisk studie (Consumption of alcohol beverages in Sweden 1920–1951, an econometric study). Uppsala: Universitetets Statistiska Institution (stencil).

Clements K.W. and Johnson L.W. (1983) The demand for beer, wine and spirits: a system-wide approach. *Journal of Business* **56**, 273–304.

Clements K.W. and Selvanathan E.A. (1987) Alcohol consumption. In Thiel H. and Clements K.W. (ed.) *Applied Demand Analysis: Results from System-Wide Approaches*, pp. 185–264. Cambridge, MA: Ballinger Publishing Company.

Clements K.W. and Selvanathan S. (1991) The economic determinants of alcohol consumption. *Australian Journal of Agricultural Economics* **35**, 209–231.

Coate D. and Grossman M. (1988) Effects of alcoholic beverage prices and legal drinking ages on youth alcohol use. *Journal of Law and Economics* **31**, 145–171.

Comanor W.S. and Wilson T.A. (1974) *Advertising and Market Power*. Cambridge, MA: Harvard University Press.

Cook P.J. (1981) The effect of liquor taxes on drinking cirrhosis and auto accidents. In Moore M.H. and Gerstein D. (ed.) *Alcohol and Public Policy: Beyond the Shadow of Prohibition*, pp. 255–285. Washington, DC: National Academy Press.

Cook P.J. and Tauchen G. (1982) The effect of liquor taxes on heavy drinking. *Bell Journal of Economics* **13**, 379–390.

Duffy M.H. (1983) The demand for alcohol drink in the United Kingdom, 1963–1978. *Applied Economics* **15**, 125–140.

Duffy M.H. (1987) Advertising and the inter-product distribution of demand: a Rotterdam model approach. *European Economic Review* **31**, 1051–1070.

Duffy M.H. (1991) Advertising and the consumption of tobacco and alcoholic drink: a system-wide analysis. *Scottish Journal of Political Economy* **38**, 369–385.

Eecen A.M.D. (1985a) *Prijs-en inkomenselasticiteiten van alcoholhoudende dranken in Nederland.* (Price- and income-elasticities of alcoholic beverages in the Netherlands). Amsterdam: SWOAD

Eecen A.M.D. (1985b) *De vraag naar bier en geditilleerd. Een bertekening van de elasticiteiten over de periode 1960–1983.* (The demand of beer and distilled beverages. An analysis of price–elasticities 1960–1983). Amsterdam: SWOAD

EEC (1972) *Effects du prix et du revenue sur la consommation des boissons dans les Etats membres des Communautes, Collection Etudes No. 19.* Brussels: Commission des Communaute Europeenes.

Godfrey C. (1986) *Factors Influencing the Consumption of Alcohol and Tobacco – A Review of Demand Models.* York: Addiction Research Centre for Health Economics.

Godfrey C. (1988) Licensing and the demand for alcohol. *Applied Economics* **20**, 1541–1558.

Godfrey C. (1989) Factors influencing the consumption of alcohol and tobacco: the use and abuse of economic models. *British Journal of Addiction* **84**, 1123–1138.

Godfrey C. (1990) Modelling demand. In: Maynard A. and Tether P. (ed.) *Preventing Alcohol and Tobacco Problems*, Vol. 1, pp. 35–53. Aldershot: Avebury.

Grossman M., Coate D., Arluck G.M. (1987) Price sensitivity of alcoholic beverages in the United States: youth alcohol consumption. In: Holder H.D. (ed.) *Advances in Substance Abuse: Behavioral and Biological Research. Control issues in alcohol abuse prevention. Strategies for states and communities*, pp. 169–198. Greenwich, C: JAI Press.

Harris J.D. (1984) More data on tax policy. In Gerstein D.R. (ed.) *Toward the Prevention of Alcohol Problems: Government, Business and Community Action*, pp. 33–38. Washington, DC.: National Academy Press.

Hogarty T.F. and Elzinga K.G. (1972) The demand for beer. *The Review of Economics and Statistics* **54**, 195–198.

Horverak Ø. (1979) *Norsk Alkoholpolitikk 1960–1975.* (Norwegian alcohol policy 1960–1975. An analysis of alcohol political means and their effects). Oslo: Statens Institutt for Alkoholforskning.

Huitfeldt B. and Jorner U. (1972) *Efterfrågan på rusdrycker i Sverige* (The Demand for Alcoholic Beverages in Sweden). Stockholm: Government Official Reports.

Johnson J.A. and Oksanen E.H. (1974) Socio-economic determinants of the consumption of alcoholic beverages. *Applied Economics* **6**, 293–301.

Johnson J.A. and Oksanen E.H. (1977) Estimation of demand for alcoholic beverages in Canada from pooled time series and cross section. *The Review of Economics and Statistics* **59**, 113–118.

Johnson J.A., Oksanen E.H., Veall M.R., and Fretz D. (1992) Short-run and long-run elasticities for Canadian consumption of alcoholic beverages: an error-correction mechanism/cointegration approach. *The Review of Economics and Statistics* **74**, 64–74.

Jones A.M. (1989) A systems approach to the demand for alcohol and tobacco. *Bulletin of Economic Research* **41**, 3307–3378.

Kendell R.E., de Roumanie M., and Ritson E.G. (1983) Effect of economic changes on Scottish drinking habits 1978–82. *British Journal of Addiction* **78**, 365–379.

Labys W.C. (1976) An international comparison of price and income elasticities for wine consumption. *Australian Journal of Agricultural Economics* **20**, 33–36.

Lau H.-H. (1975) Cost of alcoholic beverages as a determinant of alcohol consumption. In: Gibbins R.J., Israel Y., and Kalant H. (ed.) *Research Advances in Alcohol and Drug Problems*, Vol. 22 pp. 211–245. New York: John Wiley.

Lidman R.M. (1976) *Economic Issues in Alcohol Control*. Berkeley: Social Research Group, School of Public Health, University of California.

Malmquist S. (1948) *A Statistical Analysis of the Demand for Liquor in Sweden*. Uppsala: University of Uppsala.

McGuinness T. (1983) The demand for beer, spirits and wine in the UK, 1956–1979. In: Grant M., Plant M., and Williams A. (ed.) *Economics and Alcohol*, pp. 238–242. London: Croom Helm.

Miller S.L. and Roberts I.M. (1972) The effect of price change on wine sales in Australia. *Quarterly Review of Agricultural Economics*, **25**, 231–239.

Niskanen W.A. (1960) *Taxation and the Demand for Alcoholic Beverages. Rand Report*, p.1872. Santa Monica: Rand Corporation.

Niskanen W.A. (1962) *The Demand for Alcoholic Beverages. Rand Report*, p. 2583. Santa Monica: Rand Corporation.

Norman D. (1975) Structural change and performance in the brewing industry. Unpublished dissertation. Los Angeles: University of California.

Nyberg A. (1967) *Alkoholijuomien kulutus ja hinnat* (Consumption and Prices of Alcoholic Beverages). Helsinki: The Finnish Foundation for Alcohol Studies.

Ornstein S.I. (1980) Control of alcohol consumption through price increases. *Journal of Studies on Alcohol* **41**, 807–818.

Ornstein S.I. and Levy D. (1983) Price and income elasticities and the demand for alcoholic beverages. In: Galanter M. (ed.) *Recent Developments in Alcoholism*, pp. 303–345. New York: Plenum.

Partanen J. (1991) *Sociability and Intoxication. Alcohol and Drinking in Kenya, Africa, and the Modern World*, Vol. 39. Helsinki: The Finnish Foundation for Alcohol Studies.

Pearce D. (1986) *The Demand for Alcohol in New Zealand*. Discussion Paper No. 86.02. Department of Economics, The University of Western Australia.

Prest A.R. (1949) Some experiments in demand analysis. *The Review of Economics and Statistics* **21**, 33–49.

Quek K.E. (1988) *The Demand for Alcohol in Canada: An Econometric Study.* Discussion Paper No. 88.08. Department of Economics, The University of Western Australia.

Salo M. (1990) *Alkoholijuomien vähittäskulutuksen analyysi vuosilta 1969–1988.* (An analysis of off-premises retail sales of alcoholic beverages, 1969–1988. Helsinki, Alko: Taloudellinen tutkimus ja suunnittelu, Tutkimusseloste n:o.15.

Selvanathan E.A. (1988) Alcohol consumption in the UK, 1955–85: a system-wide analys. *Applied Economics* **20**, 1071–1086.

Selvanathan E.A. (1991) Cross-country consumption comparison: an application of the Rotterdam demand system. *Applied Economics* **23**, 1613–1622.

Simon J.L. (1966) The price elasticity of liquor in the US and a simple method of determination. *Econometrics* **34**, 193–204.

Smith R.T. (1976) The legal and illegal markets for taxed goods: pure theory and an application to state government taxation of distilled spirits. *Journal of Law and Economics* **19**, 393–432.

Stone R. (1945) The analysis of market demand. *Journal of the Royal Statistical Society* **108**, 286–382.

Stone R. (1951) *The Role of Measurement in Economics.* Cambridge University Press.

Sundström A. and Ekström (1962) Dryckeskonsumtionen i Sverige (Beverage consumption in Sweden). Stockholm, Industriens utredningsinstitut, Småtryck nr. 22.

Walsh B.M. (1982) The demand for alcohol in the UK: a comment. *Journal of Industrial Economics* **30**, 439–446.

Walsh B.M. and Walsh D. (1970) Economic aspects of alcohol consumption in the Republic of Ireland. *Economic and Social Review* **12**, 115–138.

Wette H.C., Zhang J.-F., Berg R.J., and Casswell S. (1993) The effect of prices on alcohol consumption in New Zealand 1983–1991. *Drug and Alcohol Review* **12**, 151–158.

Wong A.Y.-T (1988) *The Demand for Alcohol in the UK 1920–1938: An Econometric Study.* Discussion Paper No. 88.13. Department of Economics, The University of Western Australia.

6

Access to alcohol, and the effects of availability on consumption and alcohol-related problems

If a thirsty citizen was to take a walk along a city road or village street in any part of the world, a variety of satisfactions or disappointments might be experienced. That traveller could encounter along some streets a bar or liquor store at every corner. In some townships or villages with a tradition of petty entrepreneurism, and possibly with home production of alcohol, our traveller may find alcohol being sold in every third or fourth dwelling. In some cities, pubs, cocktail bars, saloons, beer halls, or shebeens will abound. Alcohol may, in these circumstances, be available at any time of night or day, in every café and perhaps also in food shops and at the gas station, to young or old, and for the drunk or sober.

In other localities, the sale of alcohol may be closely restricted and the customer may need an age identity card before being sold a drink. Our traveller may walk several city blocks in the evening before finding a government liquor store, which by then has closed its doors for the day. At the extreme, alcohol may not be available at all along that street, and it will be an illicit commodity banned by law. The traveller will be offered a glass of water or juice, a soft drink, a cup of coffee or tea. Compare the experience of our traveller in a traditional Islamic village with the person sauntering through a village in a wine-producing Latin culture, and these contrasts become very evident. Differences in availability across countries, or even between different states or administrations within any one country, can be a matter of moderate variation or extreme degree. The experience of that traveller will be that physical access to alcohol can range from virtually open access to total prohibition.

Is there within these broad experiences any evidence relevant to the design of effective public health policy? The intention of this chapter is to explore the objective evidence for benefits from any measures which affect individual access to, or availability of alcohol, as instruments of public health. The research to assess every individual strategy is not as yet available, but over the last 10 or 20 years a great deal of useful evidence has accumulated.

The basic economic theory of supply and demand is discussed in Section 6.1 as an introduction to the relationship of alcohol consumption to availability. In Section 6.2, the empirical evidence on the effect of alcohol availability on consumption and alcohol-related problems, is examined in cases of 'sudden change' in alcohol supply. In Section 6.3 we will look at evidence for the public health efficacy of a broad array of individual ecological measures. The review will first discuss evidence for strategies which are most restrictive – prohibition for instance, state monopolies, and rationing. Consideration will continue with specific restrictions on the availability of specific beverage types, the encouragement of low or no alcohol beverages, the density of liquor outlets, hours and days of sale, drinking locations, regulations on minimum drinking age, and server training and server liability.

The scope of the control experiences to be covered in Section 6.3 is thus extensive and varied, albeit that these diverse strategies come to a common focus in their intention to influence the individual's physical access to alcohol. In Section 6.4, we will discuss the relevance of trade agreements and economic cooperation for alcohol regulation. In Section 6.5 we will briefly consider the relevance of this research to the public health options, with the major discussion of policy left to the concluding chapter.

This book is written for a plurality of cultures, and we are well aware that a policy approach such as prohibition, which may be viewed as anathema in one national setting, will be regarded as the favoured option in another. Thus at the start of this review it seems appropriate to make a plea for objectivity, as we attempt as best possible to discern where the weight of empirical evidence lies in an extensive and complex territory which has all too often in the past stirred divisiveness.

6.1 Economics of supply and demand

A basic tenet of economics is the relationship of supply to demand – supply is based upon demand. For most goods and services, without any government intervention, supply is responsive to the customer demand for these goods and services. In classical economic theory, supply is described as a rather passive part of the equation, expanding and contracting in direct response to purchasing activity. Economists have developed the concept of elasticity to describe the relative responsiveness of one economic factor to another (see Chapter 5, p. 110).

However, a direct and perfect relationship of supply to demand rarely occurs in the real world. When there exists a demand for alcohol, as there apparently is throughout much of the world, a supply (even an illicit supply) will be developed. In open economies, those who supply goods and services are motivated by their potential to realize a profit, and supply attempts to affect demand. This may take the form of price incentives to purchase, advertising or promotion to interest the consumer in purchasing, convenience in purchasing through longer hours of sale or more sources of supply to reduce the distance to travel for purchase, and so on. Thus, suppliers can affect demand. In short, demand and supply of alcohol can be mutually stimulating and reinforcing of one another. The form and level of alcohol availability suggests its social acceptability or appropriateness, especially to young people. If alcohol is readily available and convenient to purchase, then one is hard pressed to conclude that the young will not accept the normality of drinking.

As a result of its dangers, alcohol has been regulated in most countries so as to limit its availability and use. The purposeful alteration of price to this end was discussed in Chapter 5. Here we consider other intentional efforts to limit access to alcohol in order to restrain drinking and reduce alcohol-related problems.

The relationship of availability to use has been demonstrated also for other products with a potential to affect public health and safety. For example, handgun availability has been related to homicide rates (Cook 1979; Teret and Wintemute 1983). Unsupervised availability of cigarettes in vending machines has been shown to be related to increased adolescent cigarette purchases (Stanwick *et al.* 1987; Forster *et al.* 1989).

6.2 Sudden changes in alcohol availability

What empirical evidence exists that alcohol availability can affect drinking and alcohol-related problems? One type of evidence is provided when the alcohol supply is suddenly reduced or eliminated. There have been a number of instances in different countries in which overall availability of alcohol has been subject to dramatic changes. Strikes of retail sales workers or production workers in the liquor industry, while not purposeful social experiments of alcohol policy, do, for instance, demonstrate the impact of a sudden reduction in alcohol availability on alcohol consumption. Giesbrecht (1988) has provided a review of strike studies. It should be noted that strikes are themselves transient and consumers know that the inconvenience will eventually end.

Mäkelä (1980), in an early strike study, examined the effects of a 1972 strike in Finland which closed Finnish liquor stores for 5 weeks. Using observational and survey data and statistical records, he found that overall consumption of alcohol decreased by roughly one-third. Arrests for public drunkenness decreased by 50%, arrests for drink-driving decreased by between 10 and 15%, and cases of assault and battery declined by as much as 25%. It should be noted that bars and restaurants continued to operate during this time, so all sources of alcohol were not eliminated by the strike.

Later research from the 1972 Finnish monopoly strike found that during May 1972, total aggregate alcohol sales were reduced by 30%. An identical 30% reduction in recorded consumption was found for April 1985, as a result of the strike in that year. Just as with the 1972 strike, the 1985 strike produced a similar reduction in a range of adverse consequences (Österberg and Säilä 1991).

The most obvious effect during the 9-week long strike at the Norwegian Wine and Spirits Monopoly in 1978 was the rather rapid adjustment to the new supply conditions. Together with the use of home stocks of liquor, increases in beer drinking, private alcohol imports, and home production, were the most important sources for substitution. Because of this substitution most people did not change their alcohol consumption during the strike, and the decrease in total alcohol consumption was estimated to be quite modest, at 5–10%. However, certain types of drinkers did have difficulty in sustaining their alcohol consumption. Most indicators were strongly influenced by Skid Row alcoholics, so that admissions to detoxification centres, the use of detoxification rooms at the so-called protection homes, arrests for drunkenness, offences called 'home quarrels', number of drunks in the street, and injuries caused by falling, all showed a marked decrease during the strike. Thus, the reduction in the consumption of alcohol seems to have been most marked among the most troublesome drinkers (Horverak 1983).

During the alcohol strike in Sweden in 1963, the drinking habits of moderate users of alcohol were found to have been scarcely affected. Their consumption remained relatively low throughout the strike period. On the other hand, both the drinking frequency of 'alcoholics' and the amounts drunk by them decreased noticeably during the strike, and even their consumption of light beer decreased despite the fact that the availability of light beer was not impaired (Bjerver and Nevi 1965).

In Poland during the summer of 1980, mass strikes occurred throughout the country as manifestation of opposition to the communist government. In response to public criticism, the authorities undertook a number of measures to reduce the availability of alcohol. The network of retail vodka shops was reduced, a 50% reduction in potato production yielded less raw material for vodka, and vodka production was substantially reduced. As a result, demand exceeded supply and prices increased. All of these factors, together with others affecting alcohol consumption, produced a 24% decline in consumption. As a result, drink-driving arrests dropped by

40%, and the number of alcohol-related traffic crashes decreased by 10% (Morawski *et al.* in press).

A national programme adopted in May 1985, in the former USSR, was directed at reducing the production and retail availability of beverage alcohol. The programme sought especially to reduce the consumption of vodka and low-quality strong wines, and to increase the consumption of beer and high-quality wine, increase the share of alcohol sold through bars and restaurants, and to reduce the illegal production of alcohol. Descriptive assessment of this experiment suggested a reduction in the legal production of vodka and other spirits, a reduction in legal alcohol sales, and a reduction in per capita alcohol consumption (based upon recorded alcohol sales). As a result, traffic crashes by drunken drivers and alcohol-related traumas were observed to decline. Negative effects, however, also occurred as a result of these extreme restrictions. There was a sudden increase in deaths associated with drinking illegally produced alcohol, a black market emerged, and a shortage developed in the supply of sugar for household use because of its diversion to illegal alcohol production (WHO 1990). The Soviet campaign was seen to have failed, and by 1986 the government had ended restrictions on availability and production (Partanen 1993). Partanen concluded that the reason that the policy failed was the inability of the government to curb illicit alcohol production. Undeniably, however, the reform had positive effects on public health, as overall mortality declined and life expectancy for males increased. This was the success within the failure (Tarchys 1993). Mezentseva and Rimachevskaya (1990) found that rates of 'alcoholism' and alcoholic morbidity varied among the 15 Soviet Republics from 1970 to 1987. The lowest rates of such morbidity were found in the central Asian republics (Uzbekistan, Tadjikistan, Turkmenia) and Azerbaijan, where religious influences restrict personal consumption and alcohol supply.

The interpretation of these various studies of sudden change in alcohol availability should be approached with caution. They are reporting on natural experiments of extreme or unusual kind; however, it would though be wrong to dismiss these findings as irrelevant to ordinary conditions. When there is a sudden reduction in retail availability, alcohol problems decline, and when the availability suddenly increases or returns, problems rise. We are dealing here with extreme cases, but they speak to the general point.

6.3 The impact of ecological measures: the research evidence

A large number of studies have been undertaken which examine the basic premise that restrictions on alcohol availability can have significant effects on alcohol consumption, and on associated problems. Those studies which address the availability of alcohol have usually found that when alcohol is less available, less convenient to purchase, or less accessible, consumption and alcohol-related problems are lower. These studies are of two types: those which address restrictions on overall availability, and those examining specific alcohol policies in terms of their unique effects. Studies on specific control strategies have provided the bulk of the relevant research.

A relatively small number of cross-sectional studies have been conducted comparing cross-cultural differences in type of alcohol regulation (for instance, monopoly versus licence systems), but partly because of varying time-lag effects, such studies are inadequate to evaluate the true impact of regulations on consumption and alcohol problems. Only longitudinal studies are used in this review because these designs enable more confident causal attribution. For overviews of the relevant research evidence see Holder (1987, 1991), Smith (1988*a*), Gruenewald (1991), and Österberg (1991, 1993).

6.3.1 *Prohibition*

While total prohibition of alcohol beverages was undertaken in a number of countries in the early part of the twentieth century, some were eventually eliminated due to lack of popular support and compliance. A modern example of prohibition occurred in 1978 on the Pacific island of Moen in Truk, Federated State of Micronesia, following a public referendum. The referendum was stimulated by political action from Trukese women who were concerned by public drunkenness and violence, particularly among young men (M. Marshall and L.B. Marshall 1990). Public drinking was replaced with group drinking which was carried out in the more isolated 'bush' areas. Public support for prohibition has remained high and the dry law has been extended to several other islands. Three attempts to repeal prohibition have been defeated. Local prohibition is thus a viable option for small societies (particularly island and isolated societies), where it may produce positive and popular results.

During the period of political unrest in Poland in the beginning of the 1980s, a temporary prohibition was introduced in Gdansk in August 1980, resulting in a drop in admissions to sobering-up stations (Bielewicz and Moskalewicz 1982). Prohibition had strong support in the population because it was introduced during a political strike and seen as a reformist measure.

Prohibition is maintained in many predominantly Islamic countries such as Saudi Arabia and Iran. Other than in Islamic countries, policy leaders today are unlikely to consider such a total alcohol ban. Prohibitions can be accompanied by a substantial increase in illicit alcohol production and sales.

However, prohibition from a public health and welfare point of view cannot be viewed as an unmitigated failure. During Prohibition in America, for example, cirrhosis mortality declined by almost 50% (from 13.4 to 7.3 per 100 000), as did other alcohol-involved problems (Warburton 1932; Clark 1976; Prendergast 1987). Furthermore, there can be little doubt that during the first few years of Prohibition in Canada, Finland, and the USA, all indicators of alcohol consumption and alcohol problems reached the lowest level achieved in any period for which there are relevant data (Bruun *et al.* 1975).

6.3.2 *Monopolies*

One of the more prominent forms of government intervention into alcohol availability has been the creation of state retail monopolies. The role of public monopolies as the direct public expression of alcohol policy has frequently been discussed (Report from a Conference 1987; Kortteinen 1989; Mäkelä *et al.* 1991). There are some inherent characteristics of monopolies which appear to bear down on consumption. Any monopoly by definition eliminates competition in the alcohol market-place. In a retail monopoly operated to reduce alcohol consumption, demand is not able to stimulate increased availability and convenience via additional private alcohol sources. Thus, the number of retail outlets is not stimulated by demand (or expected profitability) in a monopolistic situation, in the same way that it would in a privatized environment or open market. As demand increases in a free market condition, other conditions being equal, alcohol outlets or supply will increase. Greater demand for alcohol (if alcohol regulations permit) can increase hours of sale, the use of credit cards, and the sale of alcohol in conjunction with other products such as food, pharmaceuticals, or gasoline, but if the government retail monopoly is uninterested in market forces, then such market responses will not come into play. The elimination of a monopoly therefore offers an opportunity to study the effect of a change in alcohol availability. Privatization of sales usually results in a greater number of outlets for off-premise sales, longer available hours for purchase, and also often lower prices as a result of commercial competition (Holder 1988).

Wine, an increasingly popular beverage in non-wine growing countries, has been shown to be sensitive to the form of retail availability. When wine stores are opened or wine retail monopolies eliminated, wine consumption increases. Since 1970, several US states and the Province of Quebec in Canada have eliminated public monopolies on the sales of wine and fortified wine. McDonald (1986) found that the introduction of wine privatization in Idaho, Maine, Virginia, and Washington (USA) increased wine consumption in three of the four states, while Smart (1986), concluded that similar liberalization in the Province of Quebec yielded no changes. More recent studies of the end of a wine monopoly in Iowa in 1985, and West Virginia in 1981, found an increase in wine consumption and also in overall alcohol consumption (Wagenaar and Holder 1991*a*). Mulford *et al.* (1992) reported contrary findings for Iowa only, but Wagenaar and Holder (1993) have raised some methodological problems with this study, including a change in data sources at the time of wine privatization.

Another form of retail monopoly found in the USA was for distilled spirits. Iowa, in 1987, was the first state in the USA to end its distilled spirits monopoly since the repeal of USA Prohibition. This produced an increase in total absolute alcohol consumption which included a 9.5% increase in spirits sales, no change in beer consumption and a 13.7% decrease in wine sales which had been de-monopolized about 2 years earlier. No changes in spirits sales were found in any states bordering Iowa (Holder and Wagenaar 1990).

One form of change in alcohol availability in a retail monopoly, is the introduction of self-service customer access in monopoly stores where only counter service was previously available. In such a situation, the customer can look at all alcohol products and make a selection from the shelves. Smart (1974) compared self-service and clerk-service liquor stores in Toronto, Canada. The self-service type had more customers, and they were observed to buy more than the customers of the clerk-service store. When interviewed, the clientele of the former more often reported unplanned purchases or 'impulse buying', and those who did so also reported a higher average consumption of alcohol during the preceding week (Smart 1974). Skog (1991) studied the effect on the sales of strong beer (above 3.5% alcohol by weight) in eight Swedish monopoly shops in the 1980s. He found a statistically significant increase in sales in only two of the eight stores following the introduction of self-service.

Nordlund (1981) examined the effect on total consumption in two towns in Norway of a net reduction of beer outlets resulting from restriction of beer sales to a few specialty beer stores. This so-called 'beer monopoly' produced a fall in beer sales, but some of this reduction was replaced by an increased sale of wine and spirits.

Monopolies as they are commonly operating at the end of the twentieth century may sometimes have changed their original emphasis on control and drinking discouragement, and become more commercially oriented. Sometimes they have been motivated to respond to consumer demand and have opened outlets to increase customer convenience. As such, they may not have reduced the saturation of alcohol outlets. However, monopoly systems are flexible instruments which can be operated sensitively in the public health interest. Putting health rather than commercialism first, they can discourage the competitive market forces, which otherwise drive alcohol sales upwards.

6.3.3 *Rationing of alcohol*

One approach to restricting personal access to alcohol as an alternative to prohibition, is rationing. In such a system, individual citizens are given a fixed allowance of alcohol, which they can purchase. Rationing is thus a control on the ability to purchase as much alcohol as one might otherwise wish to obtain. At a minimum, rationing is likely to raise the price of extra supplies for those who seek to obtain alcohol beyond their ration.

Such a rationing system was introduced in Stockholm in 1914, and in the whole of that country in 1920. Named after the physician who designed the scheme, the Bratt System specified that 1, 2, 3, or up to 4 litres of spirits could be purchased each month by citizens over 20 years of age. The individual ration was based on marital and social status. The rationing system was ended in 1955. Norström (1987) found that following the abolition of the Swedish rationing system, there was a fourfold increase in cirrhosis of the liver. Lenke (1990) found an 8% increase in assaults in Sweden following the end of the Swedish rationing system. One interpretation of these findings is that the repeal of the rationing system led to a redistribution of alcohol consumption. Since rationing targeted heavy drinkers, these drinkers were forced to use restaurants as alcohol sources, where food was served with alcohol and prices were higher. Alternatively, they had to pay high prices for illicit alcohol. This process ended with the end of rationing.

Greenland established a rationing system effective from August 1979, which specified that every person 18 years and older could obtain a sheet of 72 coupons per month. Different types of alcohol required different numbers of coupons. For instance, a beer required one coupon, but 3/4 litre of spirits necessitated 24 coupons. Schechter (1986) found that overall alcohol consumption dropped, as did drinking at home and child neglect. The system was terminated in April 1982, partly because of a large black market which had grown up in sales of coupons, and also because of poisoning resulting from home-produced alcohol. As a result, alcohol consumption jumped by 60%, as did many associated problems. Emergency room cases dramatically increased (Schechter 1986).

6.3.4 *Density of alcohol outlets*

Curbs on number of alcohol outlets and their location have been implemented in various countries, including restrictions on outlets near schools or workplaces. Early studies of density suggested that this factor had little effect on alcohol consumption. Ornstein and Hanssens (1985) found that outlet densities are determined only in response to demand. However, more recent studies utilizing multivariate econometric techniques including pooled cross-series analysis approaches, have demonstrated that geographical density does have a significant effect on alcohol sales, and we summarize this evidence below.

One group of studies has included market variables in analyses of time series (Walsh 1982; McGuinness 1983), and time-series cross-sectional data on physical availability and consumption (Wilkinson 1987). These studies, using data from the UK, suggest that availability measured in terms of outlet densities may be related to consumption, but interpretation is limited by the shortness of the series studied (at most 25 years).

Godfrey (1988) analysed alcohol sales data and indicators of availability in Great Britain. Using time-series data and recursive modelling, she found evidence that the number of outlets are influenced by the retail sale of spirits, wine, and beer. In addition, outlet density had an impact on beer consumption, suggesting a reinforcement of beer consumption via the availability of beer.

Lehtonen (1978) analysed the demand for on-premise consumption of alcoholic beverages in Finland. In addition to income- and price-elasticities he estimated an elasticity for supply factors. Half of the increase in on-premise alcohol sales from 1962 to 1977 was explained by increase in the number of restaurants (Lehtonen 1978; Mäkelä *et al.* 1991). A restrictive policy was thus able to dam up the demand for alcohol for a long time, but it found expression as a response to the increase in restaurant capacity.

A study by Wilkinson (1987), based on a relatively large sample of data from 50 states in the USA over 5 years, tested the relationship between numbers of outlets, alcohol sales, and drunken driving. The analysis suggested a small but significant relationship between these variables. Gruenewald *et al.* (1993) conducted a time-series cross-sectional analysis of alcohol consumption and alcohol outlets by type of beverage (wine and spirits) for 50 US states, 1975–1984. Beer had an insufficient time-series data base to support a complete elasticity estimation. The approach employed by these authors included analysis of beverage prices and income as covariates, as well as a subset of sociodemographic variables hypothesized to be related to consumption, and the design embraced a relatively large time-series data set. The results yielded elasticities for the response of retail sales of alcohol to outlet densities of from 0.1 to 0.3 for spirits, and 0.4 for wine: the implication of a 0.1 elasticity in this context would, for instance, be that a 10% increase in density of outlets would result in a 1% increase in consumption. These positive elasticities are comparable with those found by Watts and Rabow (1983), and demonstrate an increase in alcohol sales with increases in alcohol availability.

6.3.5 *The retail availability of specific beverages*

Restrictions on the availability of specific beverages have at times been implemented in several countries. Kuusi (1957) showed that the opening of state alcohol shops offering a broad range of alcoholic beverages in Finnish rural communities increased consumption for males by 40% and 15–19% for females. Amundsen (1967) found that the opening of a wine outlet in Notodden, Norway, in 1961, increased wine consumption, while spirits and illegal alcohol declined only slightly. Nordlund (1974) concluded that opening of off-licence monopoly outlets in Notodden, Elverum, and Älesund was not associated with changes in overall consumption, but this research has been subjected to methodological criticism as using only self-reported survey data (Ahlström-Laakso 1975).

Beverage availability can also be differentially subject to sudden changes as a result of government action, such as the imposition or ending of a ban on specific types of drink. Iceland was the first country in Europe to implement total prohibition, in 1912. While wine and spirits were later legalized, beer continued to be banned until 1 March 1989. Olafsdottir (1990) presented results concerning the ending of this restriction on one form of alcohol availability after the first 12 months of the relaxation. Surveys taken before and after the change in beer availability found that beer was added to the total consumption of alcohol for men, but substituted for wine and spirits by women. The survey found relatively small effects on self-reported spirits consumption. The increase in beer consumption was sufficient to raise total alcohol sales by one-quarter in 1989, and by one-fifth in 1990, compared with total alcohol sales in 1988.

In Finland, the sale of medium beer began in 1969 in all food stores and most cafés as part of a total revision in alcohol legislation, although it had been available for two decades in the state monopoly stores and restaurants (Österberg 1991). Recorded alcohol consumption increased in 1969 by 46% and this was entirely due to the rise in medium beer consumption. Mäkelä (1970) concluded that the number of drinking occasions in which the blood–alcohol level reached 100 mg% increased by as much as 25% in the year following these changes, and there was a substantial increase in the estimated number of heavy drinkers as well as an increase in overall consumption (Bruun *et al.* 1975).

In an experiment conducted by the Swedish Alcohol Committee of 1965, strong beer (greater than 3.6% alcohol by weight) began to be sold in grocery stores and in bars in two counties in 1967. The experiment was discontinued in 1968, 6 months earlier than originally intended, because it had caused serious consequence. In the experimental counties the consumption of strong beer increased very sharply and that of medium beer declined, while no effect was observed in the consumption of wine and distilled spirits. The net effect on overall alcohol consumption was estimated to be 5 % (Österberg 1991). Assaults were 32% higher (Lenke 1990). One age-group which took advantage of this change in availability was the 15–17 year olds. Lenke (1990) found that this was the age group with the largest increase in violent crimes. The experiment was terminated in July 1968, in response to complaints by citizens, and reports about excessive and inappropriate consumption of strong beer, especially by young people (Government Commission on Alcohol Policy 1977; and Lenke, 1990).

The introduction of medium-strength (3.6% alcohol by weight) beer in Sweden provides additional evidence on the results of changes in the form of alcohol availability. Noval and Nilsson (1984) found that total alcohol consumption in Sweden was 15% higher when between 1965 and 1977 medium beer could be purchased in grocery stores, rather than only in state monopoly stores. Following repeal of medium-strength beer sales in 1977, the conviction rates for violent crimes among this age-group decreased. Assaults for all ages were similarly responsive.

Increases in spirits availability, either in off-premise retail sales form, or in retail sale for on-premises consumption, appear to encourage consumption. For example, the introduction of spirits for sale to the individual drinker in bars, pubs, and restaurants in North Carolina, for the first time since the end of Prohibition, increased total alcohol consumption by between 6 and 8%, and alcohol-involved traffic crashes by 16–24% (Holder and Blose 1987; Blose and Holder, 1987). This was not surprising since a considerable number of alcohol-impaired drivers in North America reach such establishments using automobiles. Similar results were also reported by Hoadley *et al.* (1984).

6.3.6 *Regulation of beverages according to alcohol strength*

Increasingly popular in many countries is the retail sale of beverages which look and taste like alcoholic beverages, but which are relatively low in alcohol (e.g. less than 2% alcohol per volume) or contain no alcohol. These beverages are intended to provide the drinker with an attractive alternative with little or no risk of an alcohol-related problem.

Skog (1988) analysed the effect of the introduction of light beer in Norway in March 1985, and found a positive but not statistically significant point estimate of substitution. A controlled experiment by Denney (1993) using English low alcohol beers and lagers (0.5–1.2% per volume), found that it was not possible for people to become intoxicated with the low-alcohol beverages at the UK legal limit for driving of 80 mg% blood–alcohol concentration (BAC). Thus the availability of low alcohol beverages can perhaps in some circumstances contribute to an effective prevention strategy.

Such alternative beverages are sometimes encouraged through lower taxes and thus lower prices, and by making them more accessible by sale in private stores (if some form of monopoly exists), or by not controlling these products to the same extent as higher alcohol content drinks. For example, Sweden established alcohol beverage prices in 1992 such that the cost of beverages with higher content was greater than the cost of lower content products in terms of cost per gram of alcohol. In many countries the legal age for purchasing alcohol is lower for beer and wine than for distilled spirits (Brazeau *et al.* 1993).

6.3.7 *Hours and days of sale*

Most of the studies of changes in hours of sale or opening days for alcohol outlets have demonstrated increased drinking associated with increased number of hours, and decreased drinking with elimination of some days of sale.

Hours and days of sales have been the subject of a series of studies conducted by Smith (1987, 1988*a–c*), on a variety of such changes implemented in various cities and states of Australia (see also Lind and Herbert 1982). One descriptive study on the impact of extended opening hours for Scottish public houses and hotels has also been published (Bruce 1980). Although containing some methodological shortcomings, these studies present at least descriptive evidence for the impact of these changes upon a number of alcohol problems.

Olsson and Wikström (1982) examined the effects of an experimental Saturday closing of liquor retail stores in Sweden. They found a decline in the number of arrests for drunkenness by about 10% and also a decline in the number of domestic disturbances, as well as in outdoor and indoor assults. On the other hand, the evaluation did not demonstrate any effect on total consumption of alcohol. The evaluation of the permanent Saturday closing of liquor stores in Sweden produced similar reductions in adverse consequences (Olsson and Wikström 1984). Nordlund (1985) analysed the effects of an experimental 1-year Saturday closing in Norway for state stores. The findings were that the Saturday closings had little effect on overall consumption, and consumers adjusted to the closing by purchasing wine and spirits on other days or by purchasing beer. Nevertheless, the rate of acute alcohol problems was affected. A trial Saturday closing for 8 months of 10 Alko (monopoly) stores in Finland has been evaluated by Säilä (1978). In the trial area total alcohol consumption decreased by an estimated 3% and public drunkenness and alcohol-related violence also appeared to decrease. There was no evidence of an increase in the use of illicit alcohol in cases of intoxication leading to an arrest for drunkenness (Säilä 1978).

6.3.8 *Minimum drinking age*

This measure provides the only instance in which a specific age-group is barred from purchasing alcohol. While most counties have some regulations on minimum age of purchase, it is often loosely enforced and in some cases set quite low. The highest age in the world has recently been set nation-wide in the USA. These changes have afforded opportunity for a number of studies of decreased and increased age of purchase. These studies have generally found that a lowered age limit produced greater alcohol-involved traffic crashes for the age-groups affected by the change, while increased age limits reduced such crashes. Interestingly, few studies found that the higher minimum age always produced an immediate reduction in general alcohol consumption among the age-groups affected by the law. However, recent research has found lower alcohol consumption in the long-term (into the early 20s), among young people in North America in areas where the legal age limit has been raised by at least 1 year (O'Malley and Wagenaar 1991).

The US General Accounting Office (GAO 1987) reviewed 32 relevant studies, but many of these were judged to be of insufficient scientific quality to inform policy decisions. Of the 14 which met GAO's methodological criteria, four looked at fatal crashes across several states, and five examined fatal crashes in individual states (Klein 1981; Maxwell 1981; Wagenaar *et al.* 1981; Emery 1983; Florida Department of Community Affairs 1983; Hingson *et al.* 1983; Schroeder and Meyer 1983; Williams *et al.* 1983; Lillis *et al.* 1984; Arnold 1985; DuMouchel *et al.* 1985; Hoskin *et al.* 1986; Wagenaar 1987). Reports using data both from individual states and multiple states found reductions in alcohol-involved crashes for young drivers of from 5 to 28%. The GAO concluded that there was solid scientific evidence that increasing the minimum age for purchasing alcohol reduced the number of alcohol-involved traffic crashes for young people who are below 21 years old.

There has also been Canadian research on this topic. Alcohol-related crashes for 16–20-year-old drivers in Saskatchewan were analysed by Shattuck and Whitehead (1976). After the minimum drinking age was lowered in 1972, an increase in alcohol-related crashes was observed among this age group. Bako *et al.* (1976) found a greater than 100% increase in the incidence of auto-crash fatalities in Alberta among youthful drivers showing blood–alcohol levels of 80 mg% or more. He concluded that this increase was related to the lower minimum drinking age.

Ontario lowered the purchase age from 21 to 18 concurrent with the policy trend in the early 1970s in the USA; thereafter, Ontario experienced an increase in the incidence of alcohol-related car crashes among the young (Whitehead *et al.* 1975; Williams *et al.* 1975). Williams and his colleagues (1975) estimated that 28 additional persons died in auto fatalities in Ontario in the first year after the minimum age change. Schmidt and Kornaczewski (1975) found significant increases in the number of traffic accidents among Ontario drivers 16–19 years old. Whitehead (1977), following up an earlier study (Whitehead *et al.* 1975), found that the higher rates of alcohol-related crashes among young drivers continued over the 4 years after the age change.

Bracketing in time the 1971 lowering of drinking age from 21 to 18, cross-sectional surveys of Toronto high school students were undertaken in 1968, 1970, 1972, and 1974. The proportion of students who had used alcohol at least once increased immediately before and after the age change (1970–1972), but an even larger increase occurred between 1968 and 1970 (Smart and Fejer 1975). No comparison group was used. A study of Toronto college students found an increase in frequency, but not quantity per occasion, related to the law (Smart and White 1972).

Apart from these high school studies, the Canadian research offers conclusions very much in the same direction as the US reports.

6.3.9 *Responsible beverage service (server and service intervention)*

Intervention of this kind at the point of retail sale for on-premise outlets has been a popular alcohol policy in North America, Australia, and the Netherlands in recent years. Reviews of the impact of server intervention can be found in Russ and Geller (1986), Saltz (1987, 1989, 1993), and Gliksman and Single (1988). McKnight (1988) reported mixed feelings from a two-state pilot project in the USA. He found a positive change in server intervention with intoxicated patrons in Michigan but no change in Louisiana following server training. More recent studies of server training (Saltz 1988; Saltz and Hennessy 1990*a,b*) have demonstrated that it is most effective when coupled with a change in the serving and sales practices of the licensed establishment, and with training for establishment managers. Research supports a conclusion that changes in server behaviour can produce differences in BAC of patrons leaving licensed establishments, and thus their subsequent risk of becoming involved in a traffic crash or other alcohol-related problem.

These effects of server training have been demonstrated at the micro-level in retail on-premise establishments and usually as part of a study of such training. A recently completed interrupted time-series study by Holder and Wagenaar (1994), found that in Oregon, the one US state which mandated server training for all persons who sell alcohol, training produced a statistically significant reduction in alcohol-involved traffic crashes when at least 50% of servers had completed training.

6.3.10 *Server liability and sanctions against service to intoxicated persons*

The civil liability of alcohol retail establishments which serve alcohol to intoxicated patrons has been established in a number of countries, often based upon common law. This liability has been primarily reactive, that is, a means of legal redress after service to an intoxicated person resulted in personal loss or injury (Mosher 1979, 1987). This may for instance occur when an intoxicated driver, served by a retail establishment, crashes and injures or kills an innocent bystander. However, more recently server liability is being proposed as a preventative policy to encourage safer beverage serving practices and to prevent drink driving (Mosher 1983, 1987; Holder *et al.* 1993).

Wagenaar and Holder (1991*b*) examined effects on the frequency of injuries due to motor vehicle crashes subsequent to a sudden change in the legal liability of servers in the state of Texas. A multiple time-series quasi-experimental research design was used, including white noise and intervention analysis statistical models, on injury data from 1978 through 1988. The authors controlled for the effects of several other policy changes expected to influence injury rates in Texas, and for broader nation-wide changes in injury rates in the 1980s. Results revealed a 6.5 and 5.3% decline in traffic crashes involving injury following, respectively, the filing of two major liability suits in 1983 and 1984.

All US states have either criminal or civil sanctions against serving patrons who are obviously intoxicated. However, the effectiveness of these laws is a direct function of compliance and enforcement. Such compliance has rarely been studied. A recent study by McKnight (1992) found that compliance, expressed as frequency of service intervention or refusal to serve, increased by 37% after visits and warnings by law enforcement. This was confirmed by a drop (from 31.2 to 24.6%) in the percentage of persons arrested for 'driving under the influence' (DUI) who came from a bar or restaurant.

6.3.11 *Impact of changes in availability of alcohol on heavy consumers*

Epidemiological studies on the impact of changes in alcohol availability often report only the aggregate outcome. There are, however, some data on the differential impact on heavy consumers. So important are these results for the follow-through to policy implications, that we will attempt in this section to bring together the evidence on this particular issue. By examining a range of observations each of which might by itself be seen as pertaining only to the unusual or exotic, one can build up persuasive evidence to support the contention that generally control of physical access is likely significantly and differentially to influence the consumption of heavy drinkers. Cross-references will be given to studies which have been quoted earlier, but without repeating unnecessary detail.

First, there is relevant evidence to be gleaned from alcohol strike research (p. 127). Österberg and Säilä (1991) in an analysis of the 1972 and 1985 alcohol strikes in Finland found reductions in public drunkenness and alcoholism admissions to treatment clinics in Helsinki during the disruptions in alcohol availability. Taking another example, a 2-month long strike of workers from the Swedish retail alcohol monopoly in 1963, produced a drop in public drunkenness by 50% in Stockholm and 33% in Gothenburg. The percentage of occupied beds at institutions for alcoholism treatment declined from 92% before the strike to 68% during the strike (Medical Research Council 1965). The dramatic upheavals in alcohol availability in Poland in the 1980s which have been described earlier (p. 130) not only produced a steep decline in aggregate consumption, but first admissions for alcohol psychoses fell by nearly two-thirds, as did first admissions for alcohol dependence (Wald and Moskalewicz 1986). The common result here is that the reduction in public disturbance, crimes of violence, and alcohol-related hospital admissions, was often much more marked than the decrease in overall consumption.

Such results could be explained by the fact that it is the lower socio-economic status chronic heavy drinkers who are more affected than drinkers who have greater resources at their disposal to circumvent the reduced availability. An exception to the general rule comes from the Finnish strike in 1972, when the frequency of arrests for drunkenness of homeless chronic drinkers was reduced to a lesser degree that was that of socially less isolated drinkers (Österberg and Säilä 1991). At that time, illicit alcohol was widely used among homeless heavy drinkers in Finland, and they were consequently less affected by changes in availability of legal alcohol. For the strike in 1985, when illicit alcohol was no longer consumed, the Finnish results again fitted into the general pattern: arrests of homeless drinkers dropped much more sharply than arrests of people having a private address (Österberg and Säilä 1991).

Another line of evidence comes from the experimental Saturday closing of liquor stores in Sweden in 1981 which showed how even minor changes in availability of alcohol can have a selective effect on heavy drinkers with limited resources. Closing liquor stores on Saturdays resulted in a decrease in public drunkenness, domestic disturbance, and crimes of violence (Olsson and Wikstrom 1982; Lenke 1990). A probable explanation is that socially marginalized heavy drinkers have difficulties in planning their drinking and in stocking reserves to circumvent interruptions in supply.

Furthermore, Nordlund (1985) found that the effects of a 1-year Saturday closing of Norwegian retail monopoly stores on problematic drinkers was significant. The number of police reports on drunkenness and domestic problems on Saturdays and early Sundays decreased.

Studies which have evaluated the consequences stemming from rationing systems, or their repeal, provide a further line of evidence. Thus, the revocation in 1955 of liquor rationing in Sweden (p. 133) was accompanied by a fourfold increase in cirrhosis mortality (Norström 1987), while the ending of rationing in Greenland (p. 133) led to an increase in reported rates for violent crime, domestic quarrels, and child neglect (Schechter 1986). A further and very important line of evidence comes from the studies discussed above on minimal drinking age (6.3.8), where the results persuasively indicate that an ecological measure can avert the otherwise situationally dangerous behaviour of young people who are prone to heavy drinking. Lastly, the studies on server training (6.3.9) and server liability (6.3.10), provide evidence for another kind of strategy which can reach the heavier drinker.

In sum it is thus reasonable to conclude that a variety of ecological measures will influence the behaviour of the heavy or problematic drinker. In one form or another, this finding is repeatedly confirmed. The contrary hypothesis that control on access will merely inconvenience the moderate drinking segment of the population while the harmful drinking of the heavy consumers goes untouched, is disconfirmed.

6.4 Trade agreements and alcohol availability

Historically, restrictions on alcohol availability and retail access (as discussed previously) are internal, not international. In most countries, the alcohol produced in that country is consumed there, but there are countries which have unique interests in international sales such as Scotland (whisky) and France and Italy (wine), due to the large international markets for these products. Even in situations where most of the domestic production is consumed within the country, expanding trade with other countries is often a significant interest. International trade agreements, such as the North American Free Trade Agreement (NAFTA) between Canada, the USA, and Mexico, or economic cooperatives such as the European Community (EC), have potential effects on alcohol policy. These issues are discussed by Tigerstedt (1990) and by Ferris *et al.* (1993).

As a result of reduced barriers or taxes on imported goods including alcohol, and to the degree that imported alcohol is not substituting for domestically produced alcohol, total consumption can be increased.

Importing alcohol without barriers can cause reductions in alcohol price as a result of competition with domestic production, or add to existing consumer preferences in terms of the types of new alcohol to be consumed.

Trade agreements and economic cooperatives can also force existing internal alcohol restrictions to be changed or even eliminated. For example, the EC has a requirement that no products from member countries can be discriminated against by any other member states. This could be interpreted to mean that no internal restrictions on alcohol availability can be applied to alcohol imported from other members. For example, this is a problem which may arise for Sweden, Norway, and Finland, which have applied for EC membership but which have long traditions of state monopolies. One interpretation of their potential membership in the EC would be abolition of these monopolies (Tigerstedt 1990). In trade agreements alcohol is most often treated in the same way as any other commodity, with concern for economic issues not balanced with public health and safety concerns. While economic interests are primary in such agreements, there is good reason to consider their potential effect on alcohol consumption and the associated alcohol problems which may result.

6.6 A confluence of evidence

Bruun *et al*. (1975) concluded that environmental controls on alcohol avail-ability can affect alcohol use and thus alcohol problems, as a part of a public policy of health and safety. In the 20 years since that publication, a large number of studies have been undertaken which test this conclusion. The weight of the empirical evidence has supported the argument that limitation on the availability of alcohol can be an effective part of a public health approach to reduce alcohol consumption, and thus to alleviate problems associated with alcohol. While many of these policies are established at state and national levels, others can be established at the community level. The counter argument to the effectiveness of alcohol availability restriction, that 'people will obtain alcohol no matter the difficulty, particularly heavy drinkers', is, on the showing of the empirical evidence, not valid. Let's sum up some of the conclusions relating to the specifics.

1. Form of retail availability. Wine has become an increasingly popular beverage in non-wine growing countries and has been shown to be quite sensitive to the form of retail availability. When wine stores are opened or wine retail monopolies eliminated, wine consumption increases. Some countries have developed a national or regional policy to increase wine consumption, in order to reduce spirits consumption. However, in general

the increased retail availability of wine appears to produce an overall net increase in alcohol consumption, even though some substitution can occur.

Changes in spirits availability either from off-premise retail sales or in retail sale for on-premise consumption, increase consumption. The introduction of spirits' sales by-the-individual-drink in on-premise establishments in North Carolina for the first time since the end of Prohibition, increased alcohol-involved traffic crashes. This is not surprising since a considerable number of alcohol-impaired drivers in North America reach such establishments using automobiles. In general, the evidence supports the potential of retail monopolies, if operated for public health, to reduce consumption and alcohol-related problems.

2. Alcohol content of beverages. The introduction of medium or high alcohol content beer in countries such as Sweden, Norway, and Finland appears to be related to an increase in beer consumption. Low- or no-alcohol content alcohol reduces the opportunity to reach high blood–alcohol levels.

3. Density of alcohol outlets. Early studies of density suggested that this factor had little effect (or mixed effects), on alcohol consumption. However, more recent studies have demonstrated that geographical density does have a significant positive effect on alcohol sales.

4. Minimum drinking age. Uniformly, studies have found that lowered age produced more alcohol-involved traffic crashes for the age-groups affected by the change, while increased age limits reduced such crashes.

5. Responsible beverage service. Such interventions have been shown to reduce the alcohol impairment levels of customers leaving bars and restaurants, and the number of alcohol-involved traffic crashes.

6. Server liability. The civil liability of alcohol retail establishments established in a few countries has been primarily reactive, as a means of redress after service to an intoxicated person results in a personal loss or injury. However, more recently it has been proposed as a preventative policy to encourage (and reward) safer beverage serving practices. One study has found lower incidence of crashes after increased liability.

7. Hours and days of sale. Most of the studies of changes in hours of sale and opening days for alcohol outlets have demonstrated increased drinking associated with increased number of hours, and decreased drinking with elimination of days of sale together with associated changes in alcohol problems.

Standing back from all this detail, what can one broadly conclude? Research findings on the relationship between alcohol availability and alcohol-involved problems which are confirmed for more than one country, certainly support the conclusion that such findings are not culturally unique – they are generalizable. On the other hand, we need to recognize that the effectiveness or ineffectiveness of any of the strategies which can affect alcohol availability is related to several interactive factors. These include public support and compliance, and the history of alcohol policy in that country. Without sufficient popular support, enforcement and maintenance of any restriction is handicapped, and means to circumvent the restriction are likely to develop. Many types of restriction will, however, produce public health benefit if there is a tradition of public support. Further limitations on retail supply in an environment where alcohol is already restricted may have less effect on alcohol problems than in a baseline situation of widespread and convenient retail availability, provided that public acceptance can be secured.

In sum the final conclusion must surely be that there is strong and diverse evidence to support the contention that policies which influence environmental access to alcohol in the street which our hypothetical traveller walks down, can support the intentions of public health, provided only that these policies are in tune with popular sentiment.

References

Ahlström-Laasko S. (1975) Drinking habits among alcoholics. *The Finnish Foundation for Alcohol Studies*, Vol. 21. Helsinki: Forssa.

Amundsen A. (1967) Hva skjer når et vinutsalg åpnes? (What happens when a wine outlet is opened?) *Norsk Tidsskrift om Alkoholsp rsmålet* **19**, 65–82.

Arnold R.D. (1985) *Effect of Raising the Legal Drinking Age on Driver Involvement in Fatal Crashes: The Experience of Thirteen States*. Washington, DC: National Center for Statistics and Analysis.

Bako G., MacKenzie W.C., and Smith E.S.O. (1976) The effect of legislated lowering of the drinking age on total highway accidents among young drivers in Alberta, 1970–1972. *Canadian Journal of Public Health* **67**: 161–163.

Bielewicz A. and Moskalewicz J. (1982) Temporary prohibition: The Gdansk experience, August 1980. *Contemporary Drug Problems* **11**, 367–381.

Bjerver K. and Nevi A. (1965) *Alkoholkonsumptionens förendringar våren 1963 hos måttliga alkoholförtärare och hos personer med alkoholproblem*, pp. 41–47. (Changes in alcohol consumption in the spring of 1963 among moderate drinkers and persons with an alcohol problem) in Alkoholfonflikten 1963, Medicinska verkningar. Informationskonferens anordnad på Wenner-Gren Center av Statens Medicinska Forskningsråd. Stockholm.

Blose J.O. and Holder H.D. (1987) Liquor-by-the-drink and alcohol-related traffic crashes: A natural experiment using time-series analysis. *Journal of Studies on Alcohol* **48**, 52–60.

Brazeau R., Burr N., Dewar M., and Collins H. (ed.) (1993) *International Survey of Alcoholic Beverage Taxation and Control Policies* 8th edn. Ottawa: Brewers Association of Canada.

Bruce D. (1980) Changes in Scottish drinking habits and behaviour following the extension of permitted evening opening hours. *Health Bulletin* **38**, 133–137.

Bruun K., Edwards G., Lumio M., Mäkelä K., Pan L., Popham R.E., *et al.* (1975) Alcohol control policies in public health perspective. *The Finnish Foundation for Alcohol Studies*, Vol. 25. Helsinki: Forssa.

Clark N.H. (1976) *Deliver us from Evil: An Interpretation of American Prohibition.* New York: Norton.

'Communities mobilize to rescue the parks' (1991) *Prevention File: Alcohol, Tobacco and Other Drugs*, pp. 7–8, Winter. San Diego County Edition, UCSD Extension, University of San Diego, California.

Cook P.J. (1979) The effect of gun availability on robbery and murder: a cross section study bof fifty cities. In : Haveman R.H. and Zeller B.B. (ed.) *Policy Studies Review Annual*, Vol. 3, pp. 743–781. Beverly Hills, CA: SAGE.

Denney (1993) Low alcohol beers and lagers and blood alcohol levels. In: Utzelmann H.D., Berghaus G., and Kroj G. (ed.) *Alcohol, Drugs and Traffic Safety – T92: Band 3*, pp. 1506–1512. Proceedings of the 12th International Conference on Alcohol, Drugs and Traffic Safety. September 20–October 2, 1992. Cologne, Germany.

DuMouchel W.A., Williams A.F., and Zador, P. (1985) *Raising the Alcohol Purchase Age: Its Effects on Fatal Motor Crashes in 26 States*. Washington, DC: Insurance Institute for Highway Safety.

Emery J. (1983) *Young Drinking Drivers Involved in Fatal Crashes. Statewide Problem Identification for F.Y. 1984 Highway Safety Plan*. Des Moines, IA: Governor's Highway Safety Office.

Ferris J., Room R. and Giesbrecht N. (1993) Public health interests in trade agreements on alcoholic beverages in North America. Paper presented at Kettil Bruun Society Meeting. June 1993, Krakow, Poland.

Florida Department of Community Affairs, Bureau of Highway Safety. (1983) *Relation of the Legal Drinking Age to Young Driver's Involvement in Traffic Accidents*. Tallahassee, FL.

Forster J.L., Klepp K.-I. and Jeffrey R.W. (1989) Sources of cigarettes for tenth graders in two Minnesota cities. *Health Education Research*, **4(1)**, 145–50.

Giesbrecht N. (1988) *'Strikes' as natural experiments: Their relevance to drinking patterns and complications, and availability and prevention issues*. Paper presented at a meeting of the Kettil Bruun Society for Social and Epidemiological Research on Alcohol, Berkeley, CA, June 5–11, 1988.

Giesbrecht N. and Douglas R.R. (1990) The demonstration project and comprehensive community programming: Dilemmas in preventing alcohol-related problems. Presented at the International Conference on Evaluating Community Prevention Strategies: Alcohol and Other Drugs, San Diego, CA, January 11–13, 1990.

Gliksman L. and Single, E. (1988) A field evaluation of a server intervention program: Accommodating reality. Paper presented at the Canadian Evaluation Society Meetings, Montreal, Canada.

Godfrey C. (1988) Licensing and the demand for alcohol. *Applied Economics*, **20**, 1541–1558.

Governmental Commission on Alcohol Policy (1977). *Alcohol Policy*. Stockholm: The Ministry of Finance. (Report SOV 1976. In Swedish.)

Gruenewald P.J. (1991) Alcohol problems and the control of availability: Theoretical and empirical Issues. Presented at Berkeley, CA, Prevention Research Center.

Gruenewald P.J. (1993) Alcohol problems and the control of availability: Theoretical and empirical issues. In: Hilton M.E. and Bloss G. (ed.) *Economics and the Prevention of Alcohol-Related Problems*, pp. 59–60. NIAAA Research Monograph No. 25, Bethesda, MD: US Government Printing Office.

Gruenewald P.J., Ponicki, W.B., and Holder, H.D. (1993) The relationship of outlet densities to alcohol consumption: A time series cross-sectional analysis. *Alcoholism: Clinical and Experimental Research*, **17(1)**, 38–47.

Hingson R.W., Scotch, N. Mangione T., Meyers A., Glantz L., Heeren T., *et al.* (1983) Impact of legislation raising the legal drinking age in Massachusetts from 18 to 20. *American Journal of Public Health* **73**, 163–170.

Hoadley J.F., Fuchs, B.C., and Holder, H.D. (1984). The effect of alcohol beverage restrictions on consumption: a 25-year longitudinal analysis. *American Journal of Drug Alcohol Abuse* **10**, 375–401.

Holder H.D. (ed.) (1987) *Control Issues in Alcohol Abuse Prevention: Strategies for States and Communities*. Greenwich, CT: JAI Press.

Holder H.D. (1988) Privatization of alcoholic beverage control: A case study from the State of Iowa, USA. Paper presented at Kettil Bruun Society 1988 Annual Meeting, Berkeley, CA, June 5–11, 1988.

Holder H.D. (1991). Alcohol policy and the reduction of alcohol problems. Paper presented at the 36th International Institute on the Prevention and Treatment of Alcoholism, Stockholm, Sweden, June 3, 1991.

Holder H.D. and Blose, J.O. (1987) Impact of changes in distilled spirits availability on apparent consumption: A time series analysis of liquor-by-the-drink. *British Journal of Addiction* **82**, 623–631.

Holder H.D., Janes K., Mosher J., Saltz R., Spurr S., and Wagenaar A.C. (1993) Alcoholic beverage server liability and the reduction of alcohol-involved problems. *Journal of Studies on Alcohol*, **54**, 23–36.

Holder H.D. and Wagenaar A.C. (1990) Effects of the elimination of a state monopoly on distilled spirits' retail sales: A time-series analysis of Iowa. *British Journal of Addiction* **85**, 1615–1625.

Holder H.D. and Wagenaar A.C. (1994) Mandated server training and the reduction of alcohol-involved traffic crashes: A time series analysis in the state of Oregon. *Accident Analysis & Prevention*, **26**, 89–94.

Horverak O. (1983) The 1978 strike at the Norwegian wine and spirits monopoly. *British Journal of Addiction* **78**, 51–66.

Hoskin A.F. Yalund-Mathrews, D., and Carraro B.A. (1986) The effect of raising the legal minimum drinking age on fatal crashes in ten states. *Journal of Safety Research* 17, 117–121.

Klein T.M. (1981) *The Effect of Raising the Minimum Legal Drinking Age on Traffic Accidents in the State of Maine.* Washington, DC: National Highway Traffic Safety Administration.

Kortteinen T. (1989) *State Monopolies and Alcohol Prevention.* Helsinki: The Social Science Institute of Alcohol Studies, Report No. 181.

Kuusi P. (1957) *Alcohol Sales Experiment in Rural Finland*, Helsinki: Finnish Foundation for Alcohol Studies.

Lehtonen P. (1978) Anniskeluravintolaelinkeinon kehityspiirteitä ja -näkymiä (Development and Prospects of the Restaurant Industry, 1962–1980). *Alkoholipolitiikka* 43, 290–298.

Lenke L. (1990) *Alcohol and Criminal Violence: Time Series Analyses in a Comparative Perspective.* Stockholm: Almqvist & Wiksell.

Lillis R.P., Williams T., and Williford W.R. (1984) Special policy consideration in raising the minimum drinking age: Border crossing by young drivers. Paper presented at the National Alcoholism Forum, Detroit, MI.

Lind B. and Herbert D.C. (1982) *The effect of 'Sunday trading' on traffic crashes.* Traffic Accident Research Unit, Traffic Authority of New South Wales, SR 82/112.

Mäkelä K. (1970) Drycesgagernas frekvens enligt de konsumerade dryckerna och mängden före och efter lagreformen (Frequency of drinking occasions according to kind and amount of beverages before and after the legislative reform). *Alkoholpolitik* 33, 144–153.

Mäkelä K. (1980) Differential effects of restricting the supply of alcohol: Studies of a strike in Finnish liquor stores. *Journal of Drug Issues*, 10, 131–144.

Mäkelä K., Österberg E., and Sulkunen P. (1991) Drinking in Finland. increasing alcohol availability in a monopoly state. In: Single E., Morgan P., de Lint J. (ed.) *Alcohol, Society and the State.2. The History of Control Policy in Seven Countries*, pp. 31–60. Toronto: Addiction Research Foundation.

Marshall M. and Marshall L.B. (1990) *Silent Voices Speak. Women and Prohibition in Truk.* Belmont, CA: Wadsworth Publishing Company.

Maxwell D.M. (1981) *Impact Analysis of the Raised Legal Drinking Age in Illinois.* Washington, DC: National Highway Traffic Safety Administration.

McDonald S. (1986) The impact of increased availability of wine in grocery, stores on consumption: Four case histories. *British Journal of Addiction* 81,381–387.

McGuinness T. (1983) The demand for beer, spirits and wine in the UK, 1956–79. In: Grant M., Plant M., and Williams A. (ed.) *Economics and Alcohol: Consumption and Controls*, pp. 238–242. New York: Gardner.

McKnight A.J. (1988) *Development and Field Test of a Responsible Alcohol Service Program.* Final Report on NHTSA Contract No. DTNH22-84-C-07170).

McKnight J. (1992) *Enforcement and Server Intervention: Report to the National Highway Traffic Safety Administration.* Washington, DC: The National Public Service Research Institute.

Medical Research Council (1965) Medicinska forskningsrdet. Alcoholkonflikten

1963: Medicinska verkninger. ('The Alcohol Conflict in 1963: Medical Consequences.') Stockholm: Norstedts. Wenner-Gren Center. Svenska Symposier.

Mezentseva E. and Rimachevskaya N. (1990) The Soviet country profile: Health of the USSR Population in the 70s and 80s – An approach to a comprehensive analysis. *Social Science and Medicine* **31**, 867–877.

Morawski, J., Moskalewicz J., and Wald I. *Sudden Changes in Alcohol Availability.* Österberg E., Giesbrecht N., and Moskalewicz J. (ed). Helsinki: Finnish Foundation for Alcohol Studies, in press.

Mosher J.M. (1979) Dram shop law and the prevention of alcohol-related problems. *Journal of Alcohol Studies* **40**, 773–798.

Mosher J.M. (1983) Server intention: a new approach for preventing drug driving. *Accident Analysis and Prevention* **15**, 483–497.

Mosher J.M. (1987) *Liquor Liability Law.* New York: Matthew-Bender.

Mulford H.A., Ledolter J., and Fitzgerald J.L. (1992) Alcohol availability and consumption: Iowa sales data revisited. *Journal of Studies on Alcohol* **53**, 487–494.

Nordlund S. (1974) Drikkevaner og vinmonopolutsalg. (Drinking habits and state monopoly sales of alcohol). Oslo: Universitetsforlage.

Nordlund S. (1981) Effects of a drastic reduction in the number of beer-outlets in two Norwegian towns. Paper presented at the 25th International Institute on the Prevention and Treatment on Alcoholism, Tours, France, 1981. (National Institute for Alcohol Research, SIFA Mimeograph No. 42, Oslo.)

Nordlund S. (1985) Effects of Saturday closing of wine and spirits shops in Norway. Paper presented at the 31st International Institute on the Prevention and Treatment of Alcoholism, Rome, Italy, June 2–7. (National Institute for Alcohol Research, SIFA Mimeograph No. 5/85, Oslo.)

Norström T. (1987) Abolition of the Swedish alcohol rationing system: Effects on consumption distribution and cirrhosis mortality. *British Journal of Addiction* **82**, 633–641.

Noval S. and Nilsson T. (1984) Mellanölets effekt pakonsumtionsuniva och tillväxten hos den totala alkoholkonsumtionen (The effects of medium-strength beer on consumption levels and the rise in overall alcohol consumption). In: Tom Nilsson (ed.) *När mellenölet försvann (When middle-strength beer disappeared),* pp. 77–93. Linköping: När mellanölet försvann.

Olafsdottir, H. (1990). First effects of beer legalization on drinking habits. Paper presented at Alcohol Policy and Social Change Conference, Norway, September 1990.

Olsson O. and Wikström P.O.H. (1982) Effects of the experimental Saturday closing of liquor retail stores in Sweden. *Contemporary Drug Problems* **XI**, 325–353.

O'Malley P.M. and Wagenaar A.C. (1991) Effects of minimum drinking age laws on alcohol use, related behaviors and traffic crash involvement among American youth: 1976–1987. *Journal of Studies on Alcohol* **52**, 478–91.

Österberg E. (1991) Current approaches to limit alcohol abuse and the negative consequences of use: A comparative overview of available options and an assessment of proven effectiveness. In: Aasland O. (ed.) *The Negative Social*

Consequences of Alcohol Use, pp. 266–269. Oslo: Norwegian Ministry of Health and Social Affairs.

Österberg E. (1993) Global status of alcohol research. *Alcohol Health and Research World* **17**, 205–211.

Österberg E. and Säilä S.-L. (1991) Effects of the 1972 and 1985 Finnish Alcohol Retail Outlet Strikes. In: Österberg E. and Säilä S. (ed.) *Natural Experiments with Decreased Availability of Alcoholic Beverages: Finnish Alcohol Strikes in 1972 and 1985*, pp. 191–202. Helsinki: Finnish Foundation for Alcohol Studies.

Partanen J. (1993) Failures in alcohol policy: lessons from Russia, Kenya, Truk and history. *Addiction* **88** (Suppl.), 129–134S.

Prendergast, M.L. (1987) A history of alcohol problem prevention efforts in the United States. In: Holder H.D. (ed.) *Control Issues in Alcohol Abuse Prevention: Strategies for States and Communities* pp. 25–52. Greenwich, CT: JAI Press Inc.

The Role of Alcohol Monopolies (report from a conference, Skarpö, Sweden, January 1987). Stockholm: Systembolaget.

Russ N.W. and Geller E.S. (1986) *Evaluation of a Server Intervention Program for Preventing Drunk Driving* (Final Report No. DD-3). Blacksburg, VA: Virginia Polytechnic Institute and State University, Department of Psychology.

Säilä S.L. (1978) Lauantaisulkemiskokeilu ja Juopumushäiriöt (A trial closure of Alko retail shops on Saturdays and disturbances caused by intoxication). *Alkoholipolitiikka* **43**, 91–99.

Saltz R.F. (1987) The roles of bars and restaurants in preventing alcohol-impaired driving: An evaluation of server education. *Evaluation of Health Professionals* **10**, 5–27.

Saltz R.F. (1988) *Server Intervention and Responsible Beverage Service Programs*. Washington, DC: Surgeon General's Workshop on Drunk Driving.

Saltz R.F. (1989) Research needs and opportunities in server intervention programs. *Health Education Quarterly* **16**, 429–438.

Saltz R.F. (1993) The introduction of dram shop legislation in the United States and the advent of server training. *Addiction*, **88** (Suppl.), 95–103S.

Saltz R.F. and Hennessy M. (1990*a*) *The Efficacy of 'Responsible Beverage Service' Programs in Reducing Intoxication*. Berkeley, CA: Prevention Research Center.

Saltz R.F. and Hennessy M. (1990*b*) *Reducing Intoxication in Commercial Establishments: An Evaluation of Responsible Beverage Service Practices*. Berkeley, CA: Prevention Research Center.

Schechter E.J. (1986) Alcohol rationing and control systems in Greenland. *Contemporary Drug Problems*, **15**, 587–620.

Schmidt W. and Kornaczewski A. (1975) The effect of lowering the legal drinking age in Ontario and on alcohol-related motor vehicle accidents. In: *Alcohol, Drugs, and Traffic Safety*, pp. 763–770. Proceedings of the sixth International Conference on Alcohol, Drugs, and Traffic Safety. Toronto: Addiction Research Foundation, Toronto, September 8–13, 1974.

Schroeder J.K. and Meyer E.D. (1983) *Influence of Raising the Legal Drinking Age in Illinois*. Springfield, IL: Illinois Department of Transportation, Division of Traffic Safety.

Shattuck D. and Whitehead P.C. (1976) *Lowering the Drinking Age in Saskatchewan: The Effect on Collisions among Young Drivers*. Saskatchewan, Canada: Department of Health.

Skog O-J. (1988) The effect of introducing a new light beer in Norway: Substitution or addition? Presented at the Kettil Bruun Society Meetings, June 5–11, 1988, Berkeley, CA, USA.

Skog O-J. (1991) *Self Service of Strong Beer in Swedish Alcohol Monopoly Outlets*. Oslo: National Institute for Alcohol and Drug Research.

Smart R.G. (1974) Comparison of purchasing in self-service and clerk-service liquor stores. *Quarterly Journal of Studies on Alcohol* **35**, 1397–1401.

Smart R.G. (1986) The impact on consumption of selling wine in grocery stores. *Alcohol and Alcoholism* **21**, 233–236.

Smart R.G. and Fejer D. (1975) Six years of cross-sectional surveys of student drug use in Toronto. *Bulletin on Narcotics* **XXVII**(2), 11–22.

Smart R.G. and White W.J. (1972) *Effects of Lowering the Legal Drinking Age on Post Secondary Students in Metropolitan Toronto* (Substudy #474). Toronto: Addiction Research Foundation.

Smith D.I. (1987) Effect on traffic accidents of introducing Sunday hotel sales in New South Wales, Australia. *Contemporary Drug Problems* **14**, 279–295.

Smith D.I. (1988*a*) Effect on traffic accidents of introducing flexible hotel trading hours in Tasmania, Australia. *British Journal of Addiction* **83**, 219–222.

Smith D.I. (1988*b*) Effect on traffic accidents on introducing Sunday alcohol sales in Brisbane, Australia. *International Journal of the Addictions* **23**, 1091–1099.

Smith D.I. (1988*c*) Effect on casualty traffic accidents of the introduction of 10 p.m. Monday to Saturday hotel closing in Victoria. *Australian Drug and Alcohol Review*, **7**, 163–166.

Stanwick R.S., Fish D.G., Manfreda J., Gelskey D., and Skuba A. (1987) Where Manitboa children obtain their cigarettes. *Canadian Medical Association Journal*, **137**, 405–8.

Tarchys D. (1993) The success of a failure: Gorbachev's alcohol policy 1985–1988. *Europe-Asia Studies* **45**, 7–25.

Teret S.P. and Wintemute G.J. (1983) Handgun injuries: the epidemiological evidence of assessing legal responsibility. *Hamline Law Review*, **6**, 341–50.

Tigerstedt C. (ed.) (1990) The European Community and Alcohol Policy (thematic issue). *Contemporary Drug Problems* **17**, 461–79.

US General Accounting Office (1987) *Drinking-Age Laws: An Evaluation Synthesis of Their Impact on Highway Safety*. Washington, DC: US Superintendent of Documents.

Wagenaar A.C. (1987) Effects of minimum drinking age on alcohol-related traffic crashes: The Michigan experience five years later. In: Holder H.D. (ed.) *Control Issues in Alcohol Abuse Prevention: Strategies for States and Communities*, pp. 119–131. Greenwich, CT: JAI Press.

Wagenaar A.C. and Holder H.D. (1991a) A change from public to private sale of wine: Results from natural experiments in Iowa and West Virginia. *Journal of Studies on Alcohol* **52**, 162–173.

Wagenaar A.C. and Holder H.D. (1991*b*) Effects of alcoholic beverage server liability on traffic crash injuries. *Alcoholism: Clinical and Experimental Research* **15**, 942–947.

Wagenaar A.C. and Holder H.D. (1993) Wine privatization in Iowa: A response to Mulford, Ledolter, and Fitzgerald with a rejoinder. *Journal of Studies on Alcohol* **54**, 251–253.

Wagenaar A.C., Douglass R.L., and Compton C.P. (1981) *Raising the Legal Drinking Age in Michigan and Maine: Final Report*. Ann Arbor, MI: University of Michigan Highway Safety Research Institute.

Wald I., Morawski J., and Moskalewicz J. (1986) International Review Series. Alcohol and Alcohol Problems Research 12. Poland. *British Journal of Addiction* **81**, 729–734.

Walsh B.M. (1982) The demand for alcohol in the UK: A comment. *Journal of Industrial Economics* **30**, 439–446.

Warburton C. (1932). *The Economic Results of Prohibition*. New York: Columbia University Press.

Watts R.K. and Rabow J. (1983) Alcohol availability and alcohol-related problems in 213 California cities. *Alcoholism: Clinical and Experimental Research* **7**, 47–58.

Whitehead P.C. (1977) *Alcohol and Young Drivers: Impact and Implications of Lowering the Drinking Age*. Monograph Series No. 9. Canada: Department of National Health and Welfare, Health Protection Branch, Research Bureau.

Whitehead P., Craig S., Langford N., MacArthur C., Stanton B., and Ferrence R.G. (1975) Collision behavior of young drivers: Impact of the change in the age of majority. *Journal of Studies on Alcohol* **36**, 1208–1223.

Wilkinson J.T. (1987) Reducing drunken driving: Which policies are most effective? *Southern Economic Journal* **54**, 322–334.

Williams A.F., Rich R.F., Zador P.L., and Robertson L.S. (1975) The legal minimum drinking age and fatal motor vehicle crashes. *The Journal of Legal Studies* **4**, 219–239.

Williams A.F., Zador P.L., Harris S.S., and Karpf R.S. (1983) The effect of raising the legal minimum drinking age on involvement in fatal crashes. *Journal of Legal Studies* **12**, 169–179.

World Health Organization (WHO) (1990) *Alcohol policies: Perspectives from the USSR and some other Countries. Copenhagen, Denmark*. Report from a conference held October 31–November 4, 1988 in Baku, USSR.

7

Public safety and drinking within particular contexts

Most of the public policy strategies described previously in this volume are those which affect drinking behaviour quite broadly. There are, however, strategies which seek to alter behaviour of the drinker within a particular context, and it is these approaches which we now consider.

This chapter will be structured as follows. In Section 7.1, the experience with drink driving countermeasures will be reviewed. Such is the extensiveness of the policy and research experience relating to this topic that the section is inevitably a major part of this chapter. However, a more general consideration of issues bearing on the same type of harm minimization approach would include boating (7.3), civil aviation (7.4), and drinking in public places (7.5), which will be considered briefly in turn. Finally, in Section 7.6 some ideas will be put forward on the overall potential for strategies which aim at this kind of amelioration.

7.1 International policy experience and research on the prevention of drink driving

7.1.1 *Setting legal limits*

As was discussed in Chapter 3, alcohol can affect motor skills, sense of balance, visual acuity, and reasoning. The level of impairment caused by alcohol varies, particularly at low levels of blood–alcohol concentration (BAC). However, laboratory tests have demonstrated repeatedly that most people show a lowered performance for response time and technical tasks as their BAC increases, sometimes even with the equivalent of only one drink, and impairment will continue as BAC declines (Mills and Bisgrove 1983; Perez-Reyes *et al.* 1988; Kennedy *et al.* 1990; Pauwels and Helsen, 1993).

Drinking can therefore increase one's risk of harm and the potential for harm to others, as a result of impaired functioning. Such harm can be immediate, and one does not have to await the end of a long drinking career to die in a drink driving accident.

A legal limit for BAC has been set in most industrialized countries for the driver on the highway. This level is established within a given jurisdiction so as to define when a driver is presumed to be dangerously and illegally impaired, even if no accident has occurred. Any designated level is based on objective evidence on risk of impairment at different BACs, but also inevitably reflects a compromise between perceived public convenience and public acceptability on the one hand, and public safety on the other. The establishment of any BAC limit and the setting of such limits at progressively lower levels, has been directly influenced by evidence on individual risk distributions for traffic crashes (see discussion in Chapter 3).

Countries have varying standards for determining legal alcohol impairment. The limit can be as low as zero or as high as 200 mg%. The BAC limit is 20 mg% in Sweden and 100 mg% in many US states. In general, as research continues to demonstrate alcohol involvement in traffic crashes and public awareness increases, BAC levels are being established in countries which previously lacked such limits, while in countries which already have such legislation in place the limits are often being lowered. In reality, a person may become impaired at much lower BAC levels than those commonly established (Åberg 1993).

Young drinkers who drive are at risk due both to their inexperienced driving and their inexperienced drinking. One logical countermeasure is therefore to establish lower levels for young drivers. Early evaluation of an Australian zero BAC limit for first-year drivers found that night-time and weekend crashes were reduced (Drummond *et al.* 1987). Hingson *et al.* (1986) found that a 20 mg% BAC limit for young drivers in Maine (USA), produced a reduction in self-reported non-fatal crashes for drivers 19 years old and younger, and reductions in rate of actual injury and fatal crashes for drivers 20 years old and younger, compared with those 21 years of age and older. A later evaluation of the Maine law (Hingson *et al.* 1988) found similar results but observed that the enforcement of the 20 mg% BAC law was sporadic, and law enforcement officers were much less likely to arrest young people than adults for drink-driving.

7.1.2 *General deterrence: level of enforcement*

A primary approach to preventing drinking in conjunction with a risky situation is deterrence. This has been a major approach to drinking and driving prevention. If there is a high likelihood that a drinking driver will be caught, and if caught the penalty is severe and quickly applied, then the drinker is more likely to avoid driving after drinking. The primary basis for this theory has been advanced by Gibbs (1975) and Beyleveld (1979*a, b*): the rate of crime (in this case drinking and driving), varies with the certainty of detection and the severity of punishment.

The general validity of this theory in relation to alcohol safety laws has been demonstrated in a series of studies of naturally occurring variations in laws or in law enforcement, reviewed by Ross (1982) and Homel (1988). These studies have also demonstrated that of the three factors underlying deterrence (certainty of detection, celerity of punishment, and severity of punishment), certainty of detection is the most effective (Ross 1982; Andenaes 1983; Homel 1988). This is especially true if the certainty is well known by drivers. There is now strong evidence for the success of general deterrence in this area (that is, deterring people from breaking the law who have not previously been caught), and the most effective approach occurs when the police engage in frequent, wide spread, and publicly visible checks along the roadway, with drivers randomly stopped and asked to provide a sample of their breath. It should though be noted that harsher penalties may result in the better financed offenders being more willing to put in a stiff defence in the courts.

While random breath testing (RBT) has enjoyed limited application in a few European countries with some success (in France, for example, as reported by Ross *et al.* 1982), Australia was the first country to implement random testing on a wide scale (Homel 1988, 1993). As a result of public pressure, New South Wales introduced RBT on a statewide basis in December, 1982. Police were required to devote at least 1 hour each day to RBT of motorists. As a result, over a million breath tests were administered in a jurisdiction with three million drivers. This high rate of testing, together with a BAC limit of 50 mg%, increased the perception of risk among Australian drinking drivers. The result was that fatal crash levels dropped 22%, while alcohol-involved traffic crashes dropped 36%, and remained at this level for over 4 years (Arthurson 1985; Homel 1988). These random checks occur sufficiently frequently in the Australian states which have adopted them that the probability of being checked during a 12-month period is one in two for a male driver. Homel (1990) observed that 'RBT in New South Wales must surely be one of the most effective drink-drive countermeasures ever enacted anywhere in the world'.

In the Netherlands, the implementation of experimental RBT in Leiden and North Brabant resulted in a reduction of drivers with alcohol in their blood systems, but especially drivers with BAC levels above 50 mg%, which is the national legal limit (Mathijssen and Wesemann 1993). In this system all drivers, or a random sample of drivers are stopped, thereby ensuring that drivers who are over the limit but show no immediately evident impaired driving will be detected, as well as those who show signs of impairment.

Norström (1983) found that although in 1976 the police in Sweden began to conduct checks, the perceived risk of such detection did not rise and drink driving arrests were not reduced. Ross (1982) in his report on the

British Road Safety Act of 1967, noted that the public were initially led to believe that the probability of being tested for alcohol and arrested was much higher than it proved to be. He stated that 'It seems reasonable to me to ascribe (the subsequent reduction in effectiveness of the law) to the gradual learning by UK drivers that they had overestimated the certainty of punishment under the law'. This finding has been confirmed by Vingilis and Salutin (1980), and Voas (1982), Jonah and Wilson (1983), and Williams and Lund (1984).

The interaction of public awareness or media profile, public perception on risk of detection, and actual enforcement, is illustrated by a research demonstration in Stockton, California (Voas and Hause 1987). The programme, which paid for 10 extra police patrols dedicated to enforcement on weekend evenings (a 10-fold increase), began on 1 January 1976. From late in 1975 to the end of 1976 the novelty of the programme produced considerable local media coverage. During this 'publicity' phase the crash rate declined by 25% as the public perception of perceived risk of arrest increased. The following year the publicity dropped off, and the driving public was left to test its expectations from its actual contacts with police on the roads. In this 'reality testing' phase the number of night-time crashes increased, but did not return to pre-programme levels. During the 'adjustment' phase spanning the last 18 months of the programme when publicity continued to be sparse, the weekend night-time crash rate levelled off at about 10% below the pre-programme period. The presence of the extra patrols had produced a reduction in drinking and driving, independent of the initial publicity (Voas and Hause 1987).

The perception on risk of detection is not dependent simply on the number of police officers devoted to enforcement, but also on the technology they employ. Checking the BAC of a driver through the use of a portable breath analyser is seen to be an effective means to detect an alcohol-impaired driver. While the police in many countries rely on observational cues, such as slurred speech, glazed eyes, or smell of alcohol, detection can be unreliable and deterrence therefore not so effective. W.N. Taubenslag and M.J. Taubenslag (1975) reported on the traffic enforcement efforts of officers in Florida where a breath test was given to all motorists stopped by the patrol after the officer had taken action on the case (traffic ticket, DUI arrest, or other citation), and released the driver. They found that only one in four of the drivers with BACs over 100 mg% were actually arrested. The others were dismissed with minor traffic citations. This result is supported by Vingilis *et al.* (1982), who found that in Canada 95% of drivers over 80 mg% (the legal limit) who were briefly interviewed at checkpoints, were not apprehended by the police.

The 'Cheshire Blitz' (Ross 1977) provides evidence on the effect of routine surveillance by police. The impact of the Road Safety Act of

1967 in Britain was restored in this one county by the chief constable who ordered his officers to breath test drivers in all accidents or when someone was guilty of a traffic offence, whether alcohol appeared to be involved or not. This policy produced an immediate reduction in serious and fatal injuries but was abandoned after a month due to public pressure. This case illustrates that police enforcement procedures such as extensive random checking of drivers are dependent upon public support. Sustained police motivation is also important, and officers who engage in successful enforcement and deterrence of drinking drivers may none the less experience disappointment due to a decrease in the numbers of drivers whom they arrest drinking (Homel 1988).

The level of alcohol impairment for commercial drivers is a specific concern in many industrial nations. Professional drivers are expected to drink little if any alcohol in conjunction with their driving. In the USA, the BAC limit for commercial truck drivers is well below the level for non-commercial drivers (Committee on Benefits and Costs of Alternative Federal Blood Alcohol Concentration Standards for Commercial Vehicle Operators 1987).

Alcohol and traffic safety is not limited to a concern about drivers. Walking when drunk can also be hazardous. A study in England found that pedestrian casualties were five to seven times as likely to have high alcohol levels as injured drivers (Everest 1993; Holubowycz *et al.* 1993). In the USA, 50% of adult pedestrian deaths have BAC levels of 100 mg% or over (Blomberg and Fell 1979). While public drunkenness can constitute a crime or a condition for police intervention in many parts of the world, rarely is it defined in terms of a specific BAC level. If the drunk is not a nuisance, he or she may be left alone. Public drunkenness laws are usually for public decorum, not safety.

7.1.3 *Deterrence of drinking–driving: punishment*

Another important part of the deterrence strategy is severity of punishment. In many countries over the past 20 years, punishment for drinking and driving has been made more severe, and the likelihood of conviction for drinking–driving has increased. Here we are talking not only about the primary prevention of drink–driving (so called general deterrence), but also about what in criminology is termed specific deterrence – the prevention of the offence being repeated.

The punishment strategy which has generally been found to be most effective has been the loss of driving privileges. Peck *et al.* (1985), in their review of the research evidence on punishment, concluded that licence suspension was the most effective sanction among those commonly used. Sadler and Perrine (1984), Tashima and Peck (1986), and McKnight and

Voas (1991), found that second drinking and driving offenders with licence suspensions had lower subsequent rates of adverse drinking incidents than did those who were referred to alcoholism treatment. Also see review by Waller (1985).

Nichols and Ross (1988), in an extensive review of the international research literature, concluded that 'licence actions have the greatest individual and general deterrent potential' among alternative sanctions. This was based upon evidence from Australia (Homel 1981), Sweden and Norway (Votey and Shapiro 1985), and the US (Tashima and Peck 1986; Zador *et al.* 1988).

If there is good evidence for the deterrent effectiveness of licence suspension, evaluations of incarceration as means of deterrence produce more ambiguous results. Nichols and Ross (1988) reviewed the international research literature and found no compelling evidence that imprisonment produces lower rates of re-arrest for convicted drink drivers. Scandinavian countries have though for over 50 years prescribed severe jail terms for drinking and driving, particularly for multiple convictions. Voas (1982) and Snortum (1984) found that Scandinavian countries have a lower proportion of fatally injured drivers, and drivers in general with high alcohol concentration, compared with most developed nations with comparable per capita driving levels. Votey (1978) used econometric time-series techniques on Swedish and Norwegian data, and found that driver fatalities were reduced by increased drinking and driving convictions. Votey and Shapiro (1983, 1985) reported evidence which supported all three types of sanctions used in the Nordic countries (jail, licence withdrawal, and fines) as effective in reducing drinking–driving.

Zador *et al.* (1988) evaluated the effectiveness of three types of punishment, and concluded that suspension of licences had the greatest effect. This study, which covered a number of US states, provided evidence of a deterrent effect for brief mandatory jail sentences for first-time drinking and driving offenders.

Snortum *et al.* (1986) reported that problem drinkers in Norway were deterred from drinking and driving by threat of jail sentence. Similar results have been found in the USA following the implementation of tougher sanctions (Insurance Institute for Highway Safety 1987*a*, *b*; Nichols 1988).

Ross (1993) has concluded that punishment, particularly severe consequences for convicted drunken drivers, is not an effective long-term prevention strategy for this population, and that effective deterrence is a preferred strategy. In general, the deterrent effectiveness of severe punishments for drink-driving conviction may be lowered if judges or juries see the punishment as excessive and are thus reluctant to convict or sentence. There is evidence that threat of jail terms can have specific deterrent impact, though this effect is probably smaller than the potential effect of licence suspension (Ross 1985; Voas 1986).

7.1.4 *Treatment for multiple drinking–driving offenders as a prevention strategy*

People who are convicted of drink–driving more than once, particularly over a short period of time, are probably heavy drinkers. As a result, treatment may be mandated by the court as a part of, or alternative to, incarceration following conviction (Ben-Aire *et al.* 1986; Bovens 1987). A brief note on the efficacy of court mandated treatment is given later in Chapter 9 (p. 194), in the context of wider discussion on the effectiveness of treatment.

The treatment of multiple drinking–driving offenders is an example of the prevention paradox. Such drivers who have high personal risks do not cause the majority of alcohol-involved problems (Perrine *et al.* 1989). Deterrence of future drink–driving across the whole population is thus the most effective strategy overall (see Mann *et al.* 1983; Stewart and Ellingstad 1988).

7.2 Designated driver

One strategy to reduce alcohol-related traffic crashes is the designation of a particular member of a group who will be drinking together, as the driver who will not drink, or who will drink only moderately. The use of the 'designated driver' is a strategy which has had popular appeal in many countries. An alternative is the safe ride strategy in which drinkers hire, or are provided with, a commercially available ride from the drinking place to their homes (Apsler 1988). Demonstration programmes to promote the designated driver approach have shown increased self-reported participation in such efforts in the USA but this increase could not be unconditionally attributed to special publicity (DeJong and Winsten 1989). Critics of the designated driver solution have suggested that it can encourage heavy and unsafe drinking among other members of the group, and can undermine non-drinking messages for young people (DeJong and Wallack 1992). There are no controlled evaluations of the effects of designated drivers strategies on reducing alcohol-involved traffic crashes.

7.3 Alcohol and boating

Boating and drinking has only in recent years been recognized as a public safety problem in countries where boating is a major recreational activity. In Finland, over half and in some locations up to 75% of fatal boating accidents, have positive BAC levels (Pikkarainen and Penttilä 1990). Boating safety among motor driven boats is therefore an issue of public concern in Finland. Of the boating operators involved in water accidents in the USA, 50% were found to have been drinking (National Transportation Safety Board 1993), and a 2-year study in the State of California found that alcohol was a factor in 59% of motorboat accidents (California Department of Boating and Waterways 1986). A main reason for drowning in boating accidents is often high BAC. In Finland, 70% of drowning cases related to boating, were at over 10 mg% (Pikkarainen and Penttilä 1991). Howland and Hingson (1988) have provided a general review of research findings on alcohol and drownings, including those from boating accidents.

Some industrialized countries have established legal BAC levels for boating operators, though typically these are higher than those established for road traffic in the same country. For example, Finnish law specifies a BAC limit of 150 mg% (compared with 25 mg% for the road), and waterside breath checks are conducted on lakes during the summer months. A similar stop and check programme has been implemented in the USA by the Coast Guard. The effects of such BAC laws on boating accidents or fatalities have not been systematically researched.

7.4 Alcohol and civil aviation

The effects of alcohol on pilot skills and performance are important (Billings *et al.* 1991). It has been estimated that as many as 30% of fatally injured private pilots had been drinking (Gunby 1984; Holdener 1993). The risk of a large-scale alcohol-related disaster is worrying for commercial aviation, and pilots are expected to be alcohol free. In the USA this is defined as no alcohol within 8 hours of a flight, with a BAC of 4 mg% or higher being unacceptable (ICADTS Reporter 1991). In Switzerland, the '8 hour abstinence rule' is cited in the flight operations manual, but no specific BAC level is set (Holdener 1993). National airlines in Europe have established a programme focusing on prevention, early recognition, and treatment of alcohol-abusing pilots (Holdener 1993). A similar programme was established in the USA in cooperation with the Airline Pilots Association. The National Driver Registry in the USA has been used since 1990 to identify and ground pilots involved in alcohol- or other drug-related offences (Sweedler 1993). Attention to the role of alcohol in fatal air crashes has resulted in a reduction of fatally injured pilots in the US who are under the influence of alcohol (Yesavage and Leirer 1986), but more controlled research is needed properly to evaluate effectiveness.

7.5 Restrictions on drinking settings

A policy to prohibit specific drinking locations has been implemented in various parts of the world. In North America this has usually been in terms of laws against drinking in public (sometimes to prevent public intoxication). More recently, prohibition of drinking in parks, recreational locations such as the beach, at the workplace, or in automobiles has been implemented as part of public safety policies.

Discussions of restriction on drinking in public locations in Canada have been presented by Murray and Douglas (1988) and Giesbrecht and Douglas (1990), where these measures are seen as a means to reduce conflict and violence in public parks, and to reduce the impairment of drivers leaving parks where drinking is occurring. An evaluation of such a municipal policy in Western Ontario was reported by Gliksman *et al.* (1990). In the experimental community there was an increased public acceptance of these restrictions and increased desire to comply with them, with no similar change in the control. These findings provide initial evidence that communities are not necessarily opposed to local policies to restrict the use of alcohol in public recreational facilities. There is as yet no controlled evaluation of the effects of these kinds of restrictions on alcohol-involved events at public locations, or on the impact for the subsequent drinking and driving by participants.

Stadiums around the world are sites for large-scale popular activities, involving many sports. These arenas are, furthermore, increasingly important sources of income, including profits from the sale of alcohol. However, pride in a team when coupled with drinking can at times give rise to rowdy, hostile, or violent behaviour. In countries where a common means to reach the stadium is a private automobile, alcohol-impaired driving can add to the possible unhappy consequences of an intended happy time out. As a result many sports arenas have banned consumption and sale of alcohol, or ended the sale of alcohol at least an hour before the expected end of the competition, in order to reduce the BAC of drinking spectators (Fisher and Single 1987; Colman 1991). The effectiveness of such stadium restrictions has not been researched.

7.6 Separating drinking from dangerous situations: lessons to be learnt and ways forward

Responses to drinking–driving are in many countries viewed today as constituting at least a partial success story. Far too many people are still killed on the roads, but the material reviewed in this chapter provides persuasive evidence to show that drinking–driving legislation, when energetically enforced, is a highly effective public policy in terms of injuries averted and lives saved. However, these advances in public policy and the public acceptance of their enforcement have not come about in a day; they have

162   *Alcohol Policy and the Public Good*

been made stepwise, and have been guided and supported by a sustained research effort.

The lessons appear to be several. One is that staying with a problem over time and making strong connections between science and policy can, with patience, give a favourable pay-off. Drink–driving enforcement is now what might be termed an 'intelligent' policy: we know it works, and have insights on how to maximize its working. Another point to be made is that one can see here an interesting example of enforcement acting in support of health interests, but with the legal provision only being feasible with public support and awareness of the risk of detection and possible arrest. Lastly, it could be argued that the drinking–driving experience points to the fact that specific interventions targeted at specific types of drinking problem can produce benefit, as well as overall strategies of the kinds discussed in several other chapters.

As for the way ahead, so far as drinking–driving is concerned, there is a clear need for continued research, further policy development, and a resolute and high profile enforcement of existing provisions. There are also interesting questions as to how the lessons learnt in relation to drinking–driving can be extended toward other types of problems. We have in this chapter mentioned several related areas where there are some beginnings of policy experience although still very little research assessment – boating, flying, and legislation targeted on drinking at public events, provide examples. There is a need for further imaginative thinking as to other types of problems where, with public acceptance, policies can be devised to separate drinking from potential danger.

References

Åberg L. (1992) Behaviors and opinions of Swedish drivers before and after the 0.02% legal BAC limit of 1990. In: Utzelmann H.-D., Berghaus G., and Kroj G. (ed.) *Alcohol, Drugs and Traffic Safety – T92: Band 3*, pp.1266–1270. Proceedings of the 12th International Conference on Alcohol, Drugs and Traffic Safety, September 28 to October 2, 1992, Cologne, Germany.

Andenaes J. (1983) Prevention and deterrence – General and special. In: Kaye S. and Meier G.W. (ed.) *Proceedings of the Ninth International Conference on Alcohol, Drugs, and Traffic Safety, San Juan, Puerto Rico, 1983*, pp. 31–40. DOT HS-806-814. Washington, DC: National Highway Traffic Safety Administration.

Apsler R. (1988) Transportation alternatives for drinkers. In: US Department of Health and Human Services (ed.) *Surgeon General's Workshop on Drunk Driving: Background Papers*, pp. 234–246. Rockville, MD: USDHHS.

Arthurson R. (1985) *Evaluation of Random Breath Testing*. Sydney: Traffic Authority of New South Wales, Research Note RN 10/85.

Ben-Aire O., Swartz T., and George G.C.W. (1986) The compulsory treatment of alcoholic drunken drivers referred by the courts: A 7 to 9 years outcome study. *International Journal of Law and Psychiatry* **9**, 229–235.

Beyleveld D. (1979*a*) Deterrence research as a basis for deterrence policies. *Howard Journal of Penology and Crime Prevention* **18**, 135–149.

Beyleveld D. (1979*b*) Identifying, explaining, and predicting deterrence. *The British Journal of Criminology*, **19**, 205–224.

Billings C.E., Demosthenes T., White T.R., and O'Hara D.B. (1991) Effects of alcohol on pilot performance during simulated flight. *Aviation Space and Environmental Medicine* **62**, 233–235.

Blomberg R.D. and Fell J.C. (1979) A comparison of alcohol involvement in pedestrians and pedestrian casualties. *Proceedings of the 23rd Annual Conference of the American Association for Automotive Medicine*, pp. 1–17.

Bovens R. (1987) Alcohol program: An educational program for drunken drivers in prison. In: Brand-Koolen M.J.M. (ed.) *Studies on the Dutch Prison System*, pp. 151–157. Berkeley, CA: Kugler Publications.

California Dept of Boating and Waterways (1986) *Boating Safety Report: A Study of Alcohol Related Accidents, Youth Operator Accidents, and Repeat Offenders.* Sacramento, CA: State of California.

Colman V. (1991) Alcohol use in large facilities: Legal and health considerations. Presented at the 68th Annual Meeting of the Western Fairs Association, January 30, 1991, San Jose, CA.

Committee on Benefits and Costs of Alternative Federal Blood Alcohol Concentration Standards for Commercial Vehicle Operators (1987) *Zero Alcohol and Other Options: Limits for Truck and Bus Drivers.* Washington, DC: Transportation Research Board, National Research Council.

DeJong W. and Wallack L. (1992) The role of designated driver programs in the prevention of alcohol-impaired driving: a critical reassessment. *Health Education Quarterly* **19**, 429–442.

Drummond A.E., Cave T.C., and Healy D.J. (1987) The risk of accident involvement by time of week – an assessment of the effects of zero BAC legislation and the potential of driving curfews. In: Benjamin T. (ed.) *Young Drivers Impaired by Alcohol and Other Drugs*, pp. 385–398. London: Royal Society of Medicine Services.

Everest J.T. (1993) Patterns of pedestrian injury accidents, and their associated measured blood/breath alcohol concentrations. In: Utzelmann H.-D., Berghaus G., and Kroj G. (ed.) *Alcohol, Drugs and Traffic Safety – T92: Band 2*, pp. 924–932. Proceedings of the 12th International Conference on Alcohol, Drugs and Traffic Safety, September 28 to October 2, 1992, Cologne, Germany.

Fisher H. and Single E. (1987) Beer in the ballpark. Presented at the National Alcoholism Forum 'Alcohol and Sports' sponsored by the National Council on Alcoholism, April 22–26, 1987, Cleveland, OH. Toronto: Prevention Studies Department, Addiction Research Foundation.

Gibbs J.P. (1975) *Crime, Punishment, and Deterrence.* New York: Elsevier.

Giesbrecht N. and Douglas R.R. (1990) The demonstration project and comprehensive community programming: Dilemmas in preventing alcohol-related problems. Presented at the International Conference on Evaluating Community Prevention Strategies: Alcohol and Other Drugs, San Diego, CA, January 11–13, 1990.

Gliksman L., Douglas R.R., Thomson M., Moffatt K., Smythe C., and Caverson R. (1990) Promoting municipal alcohol policies: An evaluation of a campaign. *Contemporary Drug Problems* **17**, 391–420.

Gunby P. (1984) Any alcohol involvement unacceptable in aviation. *Journal of the American Medical Association* **252**, 1835–1837.

Hingson R., Heeren T., and Morelock S. (1986) Preliminary effects of Maine's 1982 0.02 law to reduce teenage driving after drinking. In: Benjamin T. (ed.) *Young Drivers Impaired by Alcohol and Other Drugs*, pp. 377–384. London: Royal Society of Medicine Services.

Hingson R., Howland J., Morelock S., and Heeren T. (1988) Legal interventions to reduce drunken driving and related fatalities among youthful drivers. *Alcohol, Drugs, and Driving* **4**, 87–98.

Holdener F.O. (1993) Alcohol and civil aviation. *Addiction* **88** (Suppl.), 953–958.

Holubowycz O.T., McLean A.J., and Kloeden C.N. (1993) Blood alcohol concentrations of pedestrians admitted to hospital. In: Utzelmann H.-D., Berghaus G., and Kroj G. (ed.) *Alcohol, Drugs and Traffic Safety – T92: Band 2*, pp. 977–980. Proceedings of the 12th International Conference on Alcohol, Drugs and Traffic Safety, September 28 to October 2, 1992, Cologne, Germany.

Homel R. (1981) Penalties and the drunk/driver: A study of one thousand offenders. *Australian and New Zealand Journal of Criminology* **14**, 225–241.

Homel R. (1988) *Policing and Punishing the Drinking Driver: A Study of General and Specific Deterrence*. New York: Springer-Verlag.

Homel R. (1990) Drink–driving countermeasures in Australia. Paper presented at the International Congress on Drinking and Driving as part of the plenary session 'Drinking and Driving – A Global Perspective,' Edmonton, Alberta, Canada, March 28–30, 1990.

Homel R. (1993) Random breath testing in Australia: Getting it to work according to specifications. *Addiction* **88** (Suppl.), 27–33S.

Howland J. and Hingson R. (1988) Alcohol as a risk factor for drownings: A review of the literature (1950–1985). *Accident Analysis and Prevention* **20**, 19–25.

Insurance Institute for Highway Safety (1987a) *Drinking and Driving Down Sharply in US During Last 13 Years*. Washington, DC: The Institute.

Insurance Institute for Highway Safety (1987b) Drunk driving drops sharply across nation. *Status Report* **22** (10),4.

International Committee on Alcohol, Drugs and Traffic Safety. ICADTS Reporter (1991) Sweedler, B.M., Stewart, K. (eds.) Vol. 1, No. 4. Potomac Press, Bethesda, MD.

Jonah B.A. and Wilson R.A. (1983) Improving the effectiveness of drinking–driving enforcement through increased efficiency. *Accident Analysis and Prevention* **15**, 463–481.

Kennedy R.S., Wilkes R.L., and Rugotzke, G.G. (1990) Cognitive performance deficit regressed on alcohol dosage. In: Perrine W.M. (ed.) *Alcohol, Drugs and*

Traffic Safety: Proceedings of the 11th International Conference on Alcohol, Drugs and Traffic Safety, October 24–27–1989, Chicago, IL, pp. 354–359. Chicago, IL: National Safety Council.

Mann R., Leigh G., Vingilis E., and DeGenova K. (1983) A critical evaluation of the effectiveness of drinking–driving rehabilitation programmes. *Accident Analysis and Prevention* **15**, 441–461.

Mathijssen R. and Wesemann P. (1993) The role of police enforcement in the decrease of DWI in The Netherlands, 1983–1991. In: Utzelmann H.-D., Berghaus G., and Kroj G. (ed.) *Alcohol, Drugs and Traffic Safety – T92: Band 3*, pp. 1216–1222. Proceedings of the 12th International Conference on Alcohol, Drugs and Traffic Safety, September 28 to October 2, 1992, Cologne, Germany.

McKnight A.J. and Voas R.B. (1991) The effect of license suspension upon DWI recidivism. *Alcohol, Drugs and Driving* **7**, 43–54.

Mills K.C. and Bisgrove E.Z. (1983) Body sway and divided-attention performance under the influence of alcohol: Dose–response differences between males and females. *Alcoholism: Clinical and Experimental Research* **7**, 393–397.

Murray G.G. and Douglas R.R. (1988) Drug education – a turn on or a turn off. *Journal of Drug Education* **10**, 89–99.

National Transportation Safety Board (1993) *Recreational Safety Board Study.* Washington, DC: National Research Council.

Nichols J. (1988) *Recent Trends in the Alcohol-Related Crash Problem in the United States.* Washington, DC: National Highway Traffic Safety Administration, Office of Alcohol and State Programs.

Nichols J.L. and Ross H.L. (1988) The effectiveness of legal sanctions in dealing with drinking drivers. In: US Department of Health and Human Services *Surgeon General's Workshop on Drunk Driving: Background Papers*, pp. 234–246. Rockville, MD: USDHHS

Norström T. (1983) Law enforcement and alcohol consumption policy as counter-measures against drunken driving: Possibilities and limitations. *Accident Analysis and Prevention* **15**, 513–521.

Pauwels J. and Helsen W. (1993) The influence of alcohol consumption on driving behavior in simulated conditions. In: Utzelmann H.-D., Berghaus G., and Kroj G. (ed.) *Alcohol, Drugs and Traffic Safety – T92: Band 2*, pp. 637–642. Proceedings of the 12th International Conference on Alcohol, Drugs and Traffic Safety, September 28 to October 2, 1992, Cologne, Germany.

Peck R., Sadler D., and Perrine M. (1985) The comparative effectiveness of alcohol rehabilitation and licensing control actions for drunk driving offenders: A review of the literature. *Alcohol, Drugs and Driving: Abstracts and Reviews* **1**, 15–39.

Perez-Reyes M., Hicks R.E., Bumberry J., Jeffcoat R., and Cook C.E. (1988) Interaction between marijuana and ethanol: Effects on psychomotor performance. *Alcoholism: Clinical and Experimental Research* **12**, 268–276.

Perrine M.W., Peck R.C., and Fell J.C. (1989) Epidemiologic perspective on drunk driving. In: *Surgeon General's Workshop on Drunk Driving.* US Department of Health and Human Services. Rockville, MD:USDHHS: pp. 35–76.

Pikkarainen J. and Penttilä A. (1990) Alcohol and fatal accidents in recreational boating. A ten year study in Finland. In: Perrine M.W. (ed.) *Alcohol, Drugs and Traffic Safety: Proceedings of the 11th International Conference on Alcohol, Drugs and Traffic Safety, October 24–27, 1989, Chicago, IL*, pp. 283–290. Chicago, IL: National Safety Council.

Pikkarainen J. and Penttil, A. (1991) Alcohol and recreational boating in Finland since 1978. Paper presented at VI Nordiska Trafikmedicinska. Kongressen, Akureyri Island, Finland, 7–9 August.

Ross H.L. (1977) Deterrence regained: The Cheshire constabulary's breathaliser blitz. *Journal of Legal Studies* **6**, 241–249.

Ross H.L. (1982) *Deterring the Drinking Driver – Legal Policy and Social Control*. Lexington, MA: Lexington Books, Heath.

Ross H.L. (1985) Deterring drunken driving: An analysis of current efforts. *Journal of Studies on Alcohol Supplement* **10**, 122–128.

Ross H.L. (1993) Punishment as a factor in preventing alcohol-related accidents. *Addiction* **88**, (Suppl.), 997–1002.

Ross H.L., McCleary R., and Epperlein T. (1982) Deterrence of drinking and driving in France: An evaluation of the Law of July 12, 1978. *Law and Society Review* **16**, 345–374.

Sadler D. and Perrine M. (1984) *An Evaluation of the California Drunk Driving Countermeasure System*, Vol. 2. *The Long-Term Traffic Safety Impact of a Pilot Alcohol Abuse Treatment as An Alternative to License Suspensions*. Report No. 90. Sacramento, CA: Department of Motor Vehicles.

Snortum J. (1984) Alcohol impaired driving in Norway and Sweden: Another look at the Scandinavian Myth. *Law and Policy Quarterly* **6**, 5–37.

Snortum J., Hauge R., and Berger D. (1986) Deterring alcohol-impaired driving: A comparative analysis of compliance in Norway and the United States. *Justice Quarterly* **3**, 139–165.

Stewart K. and Ellingstad V.S. (1988) Rehabilitation countermeasures for drinking drivers. In: US Department of Health and Human Services *Surgeon General's Workshop on Drunk Driving: Background Papers*, pp. 234–246. Rockville, MD: USDHHS

Sweedler B.M. (1993) Alcohol and other drug use in the railroad, aviation, marine and trucking industries – progress has been made. In: Utzelmann H.-D., Berghaus G., and Kroj G. (ed.) *Alcohol, Drugs and Traffic Safety – T92: Band 2*, pp. 912–917 Proceedings of the 12th International Conference on Alcohol, Drugs and Traffic Safety, September 28 to October 2, 1992, Cologne, Germany.

Tashima H. and Peck R. (1986) *An Evaluation of the California Drunk Driving Countermeasure System*, Vol. 3. *An Evaluation of the Specific Deterrent Effects of Alternative Sanctions for First and Repeat DUI Offenders*. Report No. CAL-DMV-RSS-86–95. Sacramento, CA: Department of Motor Vehicles.

Taubenslag W.N. and Taubenslag M.J., (1975) *Selective Traffic Enforcement Program (STEP): Fort Lauderdale, Pasco Services, Inc*. Final Report. Washington, DC: NHTSA.

Vingilis E., Adlaf E.M., and Chung L. (1982) Comparison of age and sex characteristics of police-suspected impaired drivers and roadside-surveyed impaired drivers. *Accident Analysis and Prevention* **14**, 425–430.

Vingilis E. and Salutin L. (1980) A prevention programme for drinking driving. *Accident Analysis and Prevention* **12**, 267–274.

Voas R. (1982) *Drinking and Driving: Scandinavian Laws, Tough Penalties and United States Alternatives*. Report No. DOT HS-806 240. Washington, DC: National Highway Traffic Safety Administration.

Voas R. (1986) Evaluation of jail as a penalty for drunk driving. *Alcohol, Drugs and Driving: Abstracts and Reviews* **2**, 47–70.

Voas R.B. and Hause J.M. (1987) Deterring the drinking driver: The Stockton experience. *Accident Analysis and Prevention* **19**, 81–90.

Votey H. (1978) The deterrence of drunken driving in Norway and Sweden: An econometric analysis of existing policies. In: Hauge R. (ed.) *Scandinavian Studies in Criminology*, **6**, pp. 79–99, Oslo: Universititsforlaget.

Votey H. and Shapiro P. (1983) Highway accidents in Sweden: Modelling the process of drunken driving behavior and control. *Accident Analysis and Prevention* **15**, 523–533.

Votey H. and Shapiro P. (1985) Cost effectiveness of alternative sanctions for control of drunken driving: The Swedish case. In: Kaye S. and Meier G.W. (ed.) *Proceedings of the Ninth International Conference on Alcohol, Drugs, and Traffic Safety, San Juan, Puerto Rico*, pp. 1449–1466. DOT HS-806–814. Washington, DC: National Highway Traffic Safety Administration.

Waller P.F. (1985) Licensing and other controls of the drinking driver. *Journal of Studies on Alcohol Supplement* **10**, 150–160.

Williams A.F. and Lund A.K. (1984) Deterrent effects of roadblocks on drinking and driving. *Traffic Safety Evaluation Research Review* **3**, 7–18.

Yesavage J.A. and Leirer O. (1986) Hangover effects on aircraft pilots 14 hours after alcohol ingestion: A preliminary report. *American Journal of Psychiatry* **143**, 1546–1550.

Zador P., Lund A., Fields M., and Weinberg K. (1988) *Fatal Crash Involvement and Laws Against Alcohol-impaired Driving*. Washington, DC: Insurance Institute for Highway Safety.

8

Giving information about alcohol: effects on drinking and on the social climate

This chapter is concerned with attempts which seek in the public health interest to bring about changes in alcohol-related attitudes and beliefs, and hence in drinking behaviour. Many of these attempts use the mass media as the communication vehicle but personal communication in educational settings is also popular. In many countries such efforts use up more public funds than any other prevention efforts. The likely impact of commercial advertising and, by implication, its curtailment, will also be discussed in this chapter, and advertising is certainly an influence which 'informs' people about alcohol. These various activities, whether rooted in public health or commercial intentions, have in common the fact that they target the individual. They may, however, in addition influence the public discourse on alcohol, and have an impact on the social climate rather than directly on the drinker. Both of these areas of influence will be considered in this chapter.

Evidence on the impact of these measures on the individual drinker will be reviewed in Section 8.1, and although this is a difficult area in which to mount valid research, there can be no doubt that the scope and quality of such effort has over recent years seen promising development. That section will in turn examine the effects of commercial advertising; mass media educational campaigns; community action projects; work with small groups in educational settings; and labels on alcohol beverage containers. In Section 8.2 the social climate defined as the mix of ideas about the nature of alcohol issues and ways to curtail problems, and the possible impact of these individually focused interventions upon the social climate, will be discussed briefly. In Section 8.3 the potential policy significance of this body of work will receive preliminary consideration.

8.1 The efficacy of information strategies in the prevention of alcohol problems

8.1.1 *The effects of commercial advertising of alcohol and the curtailment of advertising*

Alcohol has been one of the world's most heavily advertised products over the past two decades (Clark 1988), despite the many restrictions placed on it because of public health concerns (Partanen and Montonen 1988). The dominant themes of alcohol advertising in the 1970s and early 1980s as described in a number of content analyses, were indirect appeals associating drinking with life-styles suggesting wealth, prestige, success, or social approval. Alcohol is depicted as a normal and desirable part of life. The brand becomes symbolically invested with the positive attributes of the wanted life-style itself (Breed and DeFoe 1979; Atkin and Block 1981). In the case of beer commercials broadcast on US television in the 1980s, images and ideals of masculinity commonly linked the product with the intended purchaser (Postman *et al.* 1988).

Alcohol advertising can exert a number of interconnected effects. Some of these serve primarily a commercial function, such as putting obstacles in the way of the emergence of new brands. Advertising is intended, in a large market-place, to differentiate brands (which in reality are often virtually identical in terms of taste, colour, and alcohol content), so as to appeal to different sectors of the market. It may reinforce brand loyalty, or recruit new users to that brand. Other potential effects of advertising, of relevance to problem prevention, include the reinforcement of pro-alcohol attitudes and of drinking or intention to drink. Alcohol advertising might increase drinking among current drinkers, by encouraging larger quantities or more drinking occasions, or might discourage drinkers from cutting down or giving up. Finally, the presence and nature of alcohol advertising might influence public policy formation.

Much of the empirical research on alcohol advertising carried out by public health researchers during the past two decades has looked for direct effects on alcohol consumption either at the individual or aggregate level. At the individual level an experimental paradigm has been used in which change in attitudes or behaviour has been measured following exposure to advertising material (e.g. Brown 1978; McCarty and Ewing 1983; Kohn *et al.* 1984; Kohn and Smart 1984; Sobell *et al.* 1986; Kohn and Smart 1987; Wilks *et al.* 1992). This approach has been criticized on both conceptual and methodological grounds (Atkin 1989, in press; Thorson in press); Atkin (in press) has provided a detailed critique of many of the studies. This experimental approach assumes a strong short-term effect of the advertising which will be measurable despite the artificiality of the situation. Measures used to assess the effect of the advertising material, such as ostensible taste testing of alcohol beverages (Brown 1978; Sobell *et al.* 1986), are far removed from real life drinking situations.

Despite these shortcomings some studies, particularly those with fewer conceptual and methodological deficiencies, have suggested some impact of advertising on level of consumption. When alcohol advertisements have been embedded in television programming and covert measures made of the amount of alcohol drunk as part of the refreshments offered, there have been measurable short-term increases in the amounts consumed although results have been mixed (Kohn and Smart 1984, 1987; Wilks *et al.* 1992). For example, in a recent study in which a natural social situation was approximated, Australian students who viewed six alcohol advertisements embedded in television programmes, helped themselves to significantly more alcohol drinks than those who viewed no alcohol advertisements. However, exposure to 12 alcohol advertisements did not significantly increase alcohol consumption (Wilks *et al.* 1992). A similar finding in which more men ordered beer immediately after exposure to advertisements but with the difference not sustained, was interpreted by Atkin (in press) in terms of cognitive response theory (Cacioppo and Petty 1979). This theoretical perspective suggests that extensive repetition of messages (such as provided by 12 alcohol advertisements in a 90-minute period), leads the receiver cognitively to attack or tune out the message.

Analyses looking for effects on behaviour at the aggregate level have been carried out using records of expenditure on advertising as a proxy for exposure to advertising. A number of methodological problems have flawed all the econometric analyses which have been carried out to date (Saffer in press). Taken as a whole the findings are inconsistent: some have found relationships between expenditure and aggregate consumption levels but many have not (Grabowski 1976; McGuiness 1980; Duffy 1987, 1991; Franke and Wilcox 1987; Selvanathan 1989; Lee and Tremblay 1992). Saffer (in press) has suggested that such econometric studies are unlikely to demonstrate clear relationships between advertising and consumption because current levels of alcohol advertising expenditure and consumption, in industrialized countries, are in the range where diminishing marginal returns on the expenditure are to be expected.

If Saffer's hypothesis is correct, a more dramatic change in advertising levels, such as an advertising ban, would be more likely to show an impact on aggregate levels of consumption than any moderate changes in levels of advertising expenditure. Several studies have examined the impact of such bans. Two were of single provinces in Canada, and the methods used could not control for advertising influences from outside those provinces. No effect of the bans were shown (Smart and Cutler 1976; Ogborne and Smart 1980). However, a major cross-national time-series study of bans implemented in a number of OECD countries during the 1970s, did show significant effects. The results were consistent in showing lower levels of alcohol consumption and alcohol-related problems, as indicated by motor vehicle fatality rate, in those countries exposed to bans (Saffer 1991). Countries with bans on spirits advertising have 'about 16% lower alcohol consumption than countries with no bans, while countries with bans on beer and wine advertising have about 11% lower alcohol consumption than countries with bans only on spirits advertising'. Motor vehicle fatalities were about 10% lower when spirits advertising was banned, and about 23% lower in countries with bans on beer and wine advertising as well as spirits. It is, of course, likely that such differences also reflect other changes in those societies, given that the social climate had reached the stage where an advertising ban was deemed appropriate policy (Young 1993; Saffer 1993).

Some investigations have used survey data and looked for a relationship at the individual level between self-reports of exposure to advertising and other relevant variables, including self-reported behaviour and cognitions. This research approach does allow for measurement of longer term cumulative effects of alcohol advertising, as suggested by the theoretical perspectives of the cultivation hypothesis (Gerbner *et al.* 1986), and social learning theory (Bandura 1977, 1986).

However, it is difficult using cross-sectional survey data to tease out the causal direction of the relationships. Three studies of teenagers and young adults have been carried out and all have found small but significant relationships between exposure to alcohol advertising and higher levels of self-reported consumption, and relevant attitudes (Strickland 1982; 1983; Atkin and Block 1984; Atkin *et al.* 1984). Beer advertisements were found to increase the consumption of beer among teenagers and young adults. Strickland's data suggested that a 5-minute increase in exposure to alcohol was associated with about a 5-gram increase in ethanol consumption per day. For example, in Atkin and Block's (1984) study of young adults, those who self-reported high exposure to beers and wine advertising drank an average of 30 beers in the previous month, compared with the low exposure group which averaged 15 beers. Consumption of spirits also varied depending on exposure to print media spirits advertising. The positive correlations found in these surveys between exposure to advertising, alcohol consumption, and attitudes to alcohol, are present when other contributing variables such as demographic factors, social influences, and exposure to other media content, are controlled.

Survey data have also been collected to investigate the impact of alcohol advertising on pre-drinkers. A recent study of United States children aged from 10 to 14 years used non-recursive modelling with latent variables to assess the relationship between children's awareness of alcohol advertising, and beliefs about drinking and intentions to drink (Grube and Wallack 1994). Children who could correctly identify more beer advertisements held more favourable beliefs about drinking, and indicated that they intended to drink more frequently as adults. These effects were maintained even when the reciprocal effects of knowledge and beliefs on awareness of advertising were controlled.

One longitudinal study to date has investigated the relationship between recall of alcohol advertising and alcohol consumption at a later age. This found a significant relationship between the number of alcohol advertisements recalled by 13-year- old New Zealand boys and their self-reported beer consumption at age 18. Frequency of drinking at age 18 was not related but those who recalled more advertising (largely televised advertisements for beer), reported consuming larger amounts of beer during their drinking occasions (Connolly *et al.* in press).

In summary, the research on alcohol advertising, which has frequently been described as giving inconsistent results with little evidence of effects on alcohol consumption (Smart 1988), has been strengthened in recent years by careful conceptual and methodological critiques (e.g. Atkin in press; Saffer in press). The cross-national analysis of advertising bans, several correlational analyses of exposure to advertising, some of the more methodologically sound experimental studies, and the one longitudinal study, available have all suggested some impact. Evidence that advertising has a small but contributory impact on drinking behaviour is therefore slightly stronger than before.

8.1.2 *Effects of mass media educational campaigns*

A strategy often employed by health and welfare sectors has been the broadcast or publication of educational messages in the mass media. As television grew in pervasiveness as a medium for information and entertainment, the use of television became increasingly popular. The initial attempts to utilize television campaigns to influence drinking behaviour, and their evaluation, appeared to assume a 'direct effects' theoretical perspective in which the mass audience which was exposed to persuasive messages or information about alcohol were expected to be directly stimulated to action (Dorn and South 1983). Subsequent campaigns have modelled specific behaviours in keeping with a social learning theory approach (Bandura 1977, 1986), and have attempted to communicate messages of relevance and value to different sectors of the audience (Ajzen and Fishbein 1975; Petty and Cacioppo 1981; Rubin 1986).

Many mass media campaigns advocate 'moderate' alcohol use. They have included: strategies for reducing intake, such as switching to non-alcohol beverages (Barber *et al.* 1989); portrayal of the negative effects of intoxication or chronic use, such as impaired sexual performance which was the subject of a French campaign (Comiti 1990); and portrayal of the positive consequences of moderate use, such as sporting ability or enhanced sexual attractiveness. Illustrative of the last approach was a Californian campaign which used paid television advertising to promote lighter drinking with a 'Winners' theme (Wallack and Barrows 1983). The authors of this study reported that in the United States context of frequent television beer advertising, it was difficult to create moderation advertisements that were clearly discriminated as such by the audience.

In the United Kingdom, and more recently in Australia, the mass media have been used to advertise specific levels of alcohol intake labelled as sensible, appropriate or even safe. In the north-east of England, for example, the mass media were used to communicate drinking guidelines in a 1981 campaign which asked 'Five pints of beer every day is too much for your own good. True or false?', and which recommended two or three pints, two or three times a week. This drinking guidelines approach is not confined to the spirits and beer drinking countries which are often more concerned with the acute effects of binge drinking, but is also congruent with the concerns held in wine drinking cultures about chronic health effects. The first French television campaigns, for example, broadcast in 1984–1986, gave the messages: '*Un verre, ca va, trois verres, bonjour les degats*' ('one glass, OK, three glasses, good morning trouble') and '*pensez au deuxieme verre . . . pour l'eau*' ('Start thinking at the second glass – think of water') (Ministère des Affaires Sociales et de L'Integration 1991)

Another common theme has been that of avoiding drinking and driving (Hewitt and Blane 1984). By the mid-1980s anti-drink–driving messages had become the most prevalent US government public service television advertisements (Atkin 1989), and were also a common theme for alcohol moderation advertising funded by the industry.

However, despite the popularity of mass media campaigns as a prevention strategy, expenditure on them has not matched commercial expenditure on alcohol advertising. Most published research has not looked for direct effects of educational media campaigns on drinking behaviour using econometric analysis of aggregate consumption data, nor sought to correlate self-reported exposure to self-reported consumption and attitudes, although one recent longitudinal study found no relationship between recall of 'moderation' advertising and self-reported alcohol consumption (Connolly *et al*. in press).

Most evaluations of the impact of mass media campaigns have, instead, typically employed quasi-experimental designs to look for relatively short-term effects of campaigns on the audience. Several reviews were carried out on the evaluations of mass media campaigns conducted in the 1970s and

1980s. They concur in finding that most campaigns showed limited effect on the recipients' beliefs and attitudes, and no impact on self-reported drinking (Blane and Hewitt 1980; Wallack 1980; Dorn and South 1983; Moskowitz 1989).

This finding has applied regardless of the approach taken. For example the US 'Winners' campaign showed no influence on concern about alcohol, nor change in self-reported drinking. Awareness of drinking levels has been increased by mass media campaigns but without any demonstrable impact on consumption (Budd *et al.* 1983; Lefler and Clark 1990).

There are a few exceptions to this general finding of no effects on behaviour. The most common have been when television campaigns aiming to prevent drink–driving behaviour have been combined with other measures such as face-to-face instruction on the use of blood–alcohol level calculators (Worden *et al.* 1989), and random breath testing (Homel 1988). Drink–driving campaigns often have a clear message, in contrast to those of moderation or responsible drinking, and this has probably contributed to their relative success (Moskowitz 1989).

Supplementation of mass media campaigns with other, more personally directed interventions, has also given some indication of capacity to effect change. For example, self-reported consumption was influenced by a television campaign which advertised behavioural techniques to cut down intake, only when this campaign was supplemented by a letter sent prior to the campaign (Barber *et al.* 1989). It is also noteworthy that this campaign modelled specific behaviours, rather than attempting attitude change. There was also some evidence of a small effect on alcohol use among teenage schoolchildren when mass media messages were combined with a school-based programme, including homework which aimed to involve parents (Pentz *et al.* 1989). Similarly, a mass media campaign which was part of a comprehensive community intervention programme, produced a reduction in traffic injury (Hingson *et al.* 1993).

Mass media campaigns can also contribute to an effect on the social climate surrounding alcohol use even when the campaigns are primarily aimed at individual drinking behaviour. An evaluation of a New Zealand campaign aimed at reinforcing 'moderation' among young male drinkers found that people exposed to the campaign were more supportive of alcohol policies on availability, pricing, and advertising, compared with residents of cities not exposed to the campaign (Casswell *et al.* 1989). A mass media campaign successfully increased awareness of, and support for, a policy on the availability of alcohol in recreational spaces in Ontario (Glicksman 1986; Douglas 1990). Mass media campaigns can provide a legitimizing umbrella for community action aimed at preventing alcohol-related problems (Grant and Room 1983).

In summary, efforts to assess the effect of mass media campaigns on drinking behaviour which have utilized quasi-experimental designs, have generally failed to detect significant effects on consumption as a consequence of exposure to these campaigns. When campaigns have been supplemented by other interpersonal and policy focused interventions, they may have contributed to behavioural change.

8.1.3 *Community organization*

Community action or community organization are purposive efforts to influence the way in which people drink or think about drinking, which take place in a community context. They are broader than interventions emanating from one source such as are carried out in an educational or health institution. Community organization instead involves alliances between several sectors and often results in a multifaceted approach. Such programmes have often been combined with mass media campaigns in order to take advantage of the complementary contributions which can be made by the agenda setting function of the mass media (McCombs and Shaw 1972), and the interaction between mass media messages and interpersonal influences (Rogers and Shoemaker 1971). They have also utilized media advocacy strategies to advance public policy initiatives (Wallack 1990). There have been a few published evaluations of such community organization efforts. One such was an evaluation of a New Zealand campaign carried out in the 1980s, employing a quasi-experimental design. The objective was to influence support for key public policies including restrictions on alcohol availability and alcohol advertising, and a pricing policy. The community action included media advocacy, public events, and building intersectoral alliances to provide a public health perspective input into local policy developments (Stewart and Casswell 1993). There was also a background mass media campaign. The community action project had an impact on support for policy as measured in general population surveys, and also on the way alcohol issues were conceived by opinion leaders (Casswell and Gilmore 1989; Casswell *et al.* 1989).

In other evaluated projects the objectives have focused on a more direct impact on individuals, using small group education in community settings (Wallack and Barrows 1983; Giesbrecht *et al.* 1990). In the Californian 'Winners' campaign, mass media messages and small group discussions were used but no changes were found in attitudes or behaviour (Wallack and Barrows 1983). Giesbrecht *et al.* (1990) reported on a community intervention in a small town in southern Ontario. The major research objective of the programme was to determine if the overall distribution of alcohol consumption in the community could be influenced by modifying the drinking habits of a significant number of heavy drinkers through one-to-one education and counselling. Other aspects sought to stimulate additional programme and policy initiatives through community mobilization and organization. The results showed that the self-reported alcohol consumption of participants in the counselling programme was significantly reduced. However, there was no significant decline in the overall amount of alcohol sold within the intervention community, nor a significant shift in the distribution of self-reported alcohol consumption in the population surveyed.

One community action project which showed effectiveness in reducing alcohol-related harm was directed at drink–driving, high risk driving behaviours, traffic deaths, and injuries (Hingson *et al.* 1993). This community intervention included: school-based education; public information campaigns; increased enforcement of drink–driving and other traffic laws; and training programmes for servers of alcohol. Overall the six community intervention cities experienced a 20% greater decline in fatal crashes, compared with the rest of the state.

The evaluation of community organization approaches is a relatively new but growing field of alcohol research endeavour. As yet, evidence for an impact on alcohol-related problems is limited, but this is a strategy worthy of further research.

8.1.4 *Programmes in educational institutions*

School-based alcohol education programmes have been a widespread and popular approach. Earlier efforts were based primarily on a knowledge – attitude – behaviour model despite the lack of empirical support for that concept (Moskowitz 1989). Subsequent approaches have included social competency training of various sorts, while also incorporating technical information about alcohol and the consequences of its use. The social influences approach has included interventions targeted at presumed influences on drinking: peer behaviour, parental behaviour, and the mass media; resistance skills training to assist in resisting pressures to use drugs; strong counter-argument or opportunity to practice alternative behaviour; and life skills training to assist students in resisting drug use (Botvin 1987; Hansen *et al.* 1988*a*; Gerstein and Green 1993). Another approach has focused less on the social–environmental influences and more on the individual's affect through self-esteem enhancement, stress management, values clarification, and decision making (Hansen *et al.* 1988*b*; Gerstein and Green 1993).

Despite the large number of evaluated primary prevention programmes in educational settings, the results to date have not given cause for optimism. Reviews by Staulcup *et al.* (1979), Goodstadt (1978, 1980, 1989), and subsequently by Moskowitz (1989), reached similar conclusions. From the literature evaluating elementary and secondary educational programme as of the mid-1980s, Moskowitz concluded as follows. First, educational programmes have largely been ineffective in preventing alcohol use; whereas many programmes were successful in increasing knowledge, very few influence attitudes, and even fewer influence consumption. Second, most studies suffered from serious methodological weaknesses that undermined the ability to make inferences about programme effectiveness. Third, most evaluations neither specified the programme's goals and objectives, nor described the target population. Furthermore, the reports provided only superficial programme descriptions and the studies did not evaluate the competence of programme implementation (Moskowitz 1989).

More recent evaluations include some which address many of the methodological problems outlined. They tend to have evaluated programmes which include the social competency approach and the affective approach as described earlier. Several meta-analyses of drug education have been carried out (Tobler 1986; Bangert-Drowns 1988; Bruvold and Rundall 1988), and these and some original studies were reviewed by Gerstein and Green (1993). This subsequent research has supported Moskowitz's conclusion that there is no consistent measurable impact of education programmes on alcohol consumption, even when large-scale social influences programmes have been carefully evaluated (Gerstein and Green 1993).

College and university students have been the focus for an increasing number of campaigns. These interventions have expanded from small group sessions where information, training, or counselling was provided, to more comprehensive or interdisciplinary programmes (Bloch and Ungerlieder 1988; Caleekal-John and Pletscht, 1984), and have included the manipulation of the contexts and procedures of alcohol beverage service (Mills *et al.* 1983). Goodstadt and Caleekal-John (1984) reviewed several evaluations on college-based interventions and reported positive effects in five. However, Moskowitz (1989) pointed out that many projects have relied on administering the programme to student volunteers who may be atypical, and the nature of the course may have been irrelevant to its success.

8.1.5 *Labels on alcohol beverage containers*

The impact of the US initiative on labelling beverage containers with warnings about the effect of alcohol on health has been assessed from survey data. Six months after the introduction of labels, approximately 25% of the sample reported having seen a label, and this was higher among heavier drinkers (who were more exposed to the label). The heavier drinkers who also drove after drinking were more likely to recall the drink–drive warning, and to report taking steps to avoid driving while intoxicated (Greenfield *et al.* 1993). The increase in self-report of taking such steps was in contrast with a decline measured in Ontario, Canada, where labels were not introduced.

Pregnant women showed some decrease in self-reported drinking 7 months after the introduction of the warning labels and this was confined to the lighter drinkers whose fetuses were not at risk (Hankin *et al.* 1993). Other studies have also examined awareness of the labels' existence; the public's perception of risk; and change in behaviour (Mazis *et al.* 1991; Mayer *et al.* 1991; Mayer and Smith 1991; Graves 1992). Hilton's (1992) review of these studies suggested that achieving awareness has not been easy although awareness rates have grown over time, and awareness seems to be greater among the targeted risk groups. Most of the evidence suggests no change in the perception of risk, and only a few results suggest behaviour change which might be attributed to the warning label.

8.2 Impact on the social climate

By social climate on alcohol we mean the mix of different ways of thinking about drinking, conceiving alcohol-related problems, and defining appropriate measures for dealing with them, which exists in a society at a given point of time and which may change over time (Partanen and Montonen 1988). The interventions evaluated in this chapter, and other aspects of public discourse on alcohol, are likely to help shape this social climate, but such effects are not readily amenable to experimental analysis.

The approaches described in this chapter are primarily directed at changing individual drinking behaviour, and have been evaluated in those terms. However, whether or not they have an impact on the people whose drinking is the target for change, they may nevertheless influence the public discourse and therefore the social climate on alcohol. For example, mass media or school-based education campaigns, if funded adequately and carried out professionally, may signal that alcohol-related harm is an issue of societal concern. Similarly, while some direct effects have been suggested, it is possible that the more significant effects of alcohol advertising are on the social climate. It has been suggested that alcohol advertising communicates a meta-message about alcohol's role in society (Postman *et al.* 1988), and in turn reduces the likelihood of healthy public policies on alcohol being implemented (van Iwaarden 1983; Farrell 1985). Liberalization in the regulations controlling alcohol advertising on television so as to allow portrayals of alcohol use in association with powerful cultural myths, signal greater acceptance of alcohol use; the converse is that interventions to increase control over advertising signal increased concern. The impact of advertising bans, as measured by Saffer (1991), and as noted earlier, may, in part, reflect the public debate surrounding the introduction of such restrictions and the fact that the social climate had reached a stage at which such actions were possible.

The impact of these interventions and other aspects of the public discourse on the social climate and consequent policy making, is not easily evaluated. Nor can the impact on the social climate be presumed from the objectives of the intervention. For example, both media and school campaigns which focus on appropriate levels of alcohol use, have been criticized as reinforcing the expectation that alcohol use will occur (Moskowitz 1989). Similarly, and as already discussed in Chapter 7 (p. 159), the mass media 'designated driver' campaigns in North America and elsewhere have been perceived as detrimental to the social climate in that they detract attention from adverse consequences of drinking other than traffic crashes (Divers and Zipursky 1993), and away from alternative, more effective problem-prevention strategies (DeJong and Wallack 1992). Expenditure on alcohol education in schools may signal public concern about alcohol, but may also communicate the message that change will be achieved through individual effort rather than through public policies.

The media are believed to play an important part in setting the agenda on any issue for policy makers and the public, not necessarily telling people what to think but rather what to think about; news coverage can stimulate discussion about an issue and legitimize policy options (Milio 1986; Atkin 1989). Recognition of this fact has led citizen advocacy groups, and also public health advocates, consciously to engage in sustained action to achieve media coverage on key alcohol policy issues. Media advocacy is 'the strategic use of the mass media to advance a social or public policy initiative' (Wallack 1990).

One or two case studies of media advocacy campaigns on alcohol issues have now been published and suggest shifts in the social climate around alcohol issues, but cannot directly relate these changes to campaigns. For example, following an intensive campaign on alcohol advertising in Switzerland, which did not result in the imposition of restrictions, the media had nevertheless created an awareness such that it was impossible to take a position on dependency problems without referring to the importance of advertising (Muster 1985). Following the tax initiative proposals in California, which took place in 1990, an extensive media advocacy campaign was seen as having contributed to a lasting shift in public opinion around excise tax (Advocacy Institute 1992).

Such interventions may therefore influence the social climate surrounding alcohol use in terms of the publicly expressed concepts of drinking and alcohol-related harm, and the factors described as likely to influence these issues. Changing the social climate may in turn change the acceptability and implementation of public policies known to reduce alcohol-related harm.

8.3 The policy leads

A range of efforts to influence individuals in order to prevent alcohol-related problems have been reviewed in this chapter. The empirical evidence for a major impact from any of these measures directly on beliefs, attitudes, or behaviour is not strong. However, there is evidence to support a contributory effect. The size and nature of the impact is likely to depend on the overall mix of the messages. Monopolization, the predominance of one message, has long been identified as a prerequisite for change to be induced by mass media communication (Lazarsfeld and Merton 1948). However, the contrast between the nature of the messages found in commercial advertising (and the entertainment media), and those communicated in mass media education campaigns and school-based education, precludes such monopolization. Furthermore, in terms of the resources expended, the commercial and entertainment messages are predominant.

The results suggest that not one of the strategies reviewed in this chapter is likely to achieve change in isolation. Where attempts to educate which employ either media or small groups settings have been supplemented with other influences, or have supplemented environmental strategies, more evidence of efficacy has been found. It is likely that this is one of the most relevant messages from this review of effectiveness – education strategies, in order to have any chance of effectiveness, need to be entwined with other strategies, especially those which more directly impact on the drinker's environment. When evaluated in isolation the popular, and often well resourced interventions of school-based education and moderation mass media campaigns, have not been found to be effective.

It is also possible that the strategies reviewed in this chapter, particularly highly visible and symbolic ones such as restrictions on alcohol advertising and mass-media educational programmes, may have their most significant impact on the social climate surrounding alcohol use rather than a direct effect on the individual's behaviour. These purposive efforts, by inserting a health perspective into the public discourse on alcohol, signal societal concern about alcohol-related problems. This is then part of the social and political context in which decisions are taken about the development and implementation of public policies, many of which have larger direct influences on drinking behaviour.

References

Advocacy Institute (1992) *Taking Initiative: The 1990 Citizen's Movement to Raise California Alcohol Excise Taxes to Save Lives*. Washington DC: The Advocacy Institute.

Ajzen I. and Fishbein M. (1975) *Belief, Attitude, Intention, and Behaviour: An Introduction to Theory and Research*. Reading, MA: Addison-Wesley.

Atkin C.K. (1989) Mass communication effects on drinking and driving. In: *Surgeon General's Workshop on Drunk Driving: Background Papers*, pp. 15–34 Washington, DC: US Department of Health and Human Services.

Atkin C.K. (in press) *Survey and experimental research on alcohol advertising effects. The Effects of the Mass media on the Use and Abuse of Alcohol* (NIAAA Monograph).

Atkin C.K. and Block M. (1981) *Content and Effects of Alcohol Advertising: Report 1, Overview and Summary*. Springfield, VT: National Technical Information Service.

Atkin C.K. and Block M. (1984) The effects of alcohol advertising. In: Kinnear, T.C. (ed.) *Advances in Consumer Research*, pp. 688–693. Provo, Ut: Association for Consumer Research.

Atkin C.K., Hocking, J., and Block M. (1984) Teenage drinking: does advertising make a difference? *Journal of Communication* **34** 157–167.

Bandura A. (1977) *Social Learning Theory*. Englewood Cliffs, NJ: Prentice-Hall.

Bandura A. (1986) *Social Foundations of Thought and Action: A Social Cognitive Theory*. Englewood Cliffs, NJ: Prentice-Hall.

Bangert-Drowns R.L. (1988) The effects of school-based substance abuse education: a meta-analysis. *Journal of Drug Education*, **18**, 243–64.

Barber J.G., Bradshaw, R., and Walsh C. (1989) Reducing alcohol consumption through television advertising. *Journal of Consulting and Clinical Psychology* **57**, 613–618.

Blane H.T. and Hewitt L.E. (1980) Alcohol, public education and mass media: an overview. *Alcohol, Health and Research World* **5**, 2–16.

Bloch S.A. and Ungerlieder S. (1988) Targeting high-risk groups on campus for drug and alcohol prevention: An examination and assessment. *International Journal of the Addictions* **23**, pp. 299–319.

Botvin G.J. (1987) *Factors Inhibiting Drug Use: Teacher and Peer Effects*. Final report submitted to the National Institute on Drug Abuse, New York, Cornell University Medical College.

Breed W.A. and DeFoe J.R. (1979) Themes in magazine alcohol advertisements *Journal of Drug Issues* **9**, pp. 511–522.

Brown R.A. (1978) Educating young people about alcohol use in New Zealand: Whose side are we on? *British Journal of Alcohol and Alcoholism* **13**, 199–204.

Bruvold W. and Rundall T.A. (1988) A meta-analysis and theoretical review of school-based tobacco and alcohol intervention programs. *Psychology and Health*, **2**, 53–78.

Budd J., Gray P., and McCron R. (1983) The Tyne Tees Alcohol Education Campaign: An Evaluation. London Health Education Council.

Cacioppo J. and Petty R. (1979) Effects of message repitition and position on cognitive responses, recall and persuasion. *Journal of Personality and Social Psychology* **37**, 97–109.

Caleekal-John A. and Pletscht D.H. (1984) An interdisciplinary cognitive approach to alcohol education in the university curriculum. *Journal of Alcohol and Drug Education* **30**, 50–60.

Casswell S. and Gilmore L. (1989) An evaluated community action project on alcohol. *Journal of Studies on Alcohol* **50**, 339–346.

Casswell S., Gilmore L., Maguire V., and Ransom R. (1989) Changes in public support for alcohol policies following a community-based campaign. *British Journal of Addiction* **84**, 515–522.

Clark E. (1988) *The Want Makers: Lifting the Lid off the World Advertising Industry: How They Make You Buy.* London: Hodder and Stoughton.

Comiti V.P. (1990) The advertising of alcohol in France. *World Health Forum* **11**, 242–245.

Connolly G.M., Casswell S., Zhang J.F., and Silva P.A. (in press) Alcohol in the mass media and drinking by adolescents: a longitudinal study. *Addiction*, **89**.

DeJong W. and Wallack L.M. (1992) The role of designated driver programs in the prevention of alcohol-impaired driving: a critical reassessment. *Health Education Quarterly* **19**, 429–442.

Divers P. and Zipursky B.M. (1993) The intended and unitended consequences of promoting 'Don't Drink and Drive' messages. In Greenfield T. K. and Zimmerman R. (ed.). *Experiences with Community Action Projects: New Research in the Prevention of Alcohol and Other Drug Problems*, pp. 59–70, OSAP Prevention Monograph – 4. Rockville, MD: US Department of Health and Human Services.

Dossier de Presse Prevention de l'alcoolisme. le 2 Decembre 1991, p. 19.

Dorn N. and South N. (1983) *Message in a Bottle: Theoretical Overview and Annotated Bibliography on the Mass Media and Alcohol.* Aldershot: Gower.

Douglas R.R. (1990) Formulating alcohol policies for community recreation faciltities: tactics and problems. In: Giesbrecht N., Conley P., Denniston R. W., Gliksman L., Holder H., Pederson A., Room, R., and Shain, M. (ed.) *Research, Action, and the Community: Experience in the Prevention of Alcohol and Other Drug Problems*, pp. 61–67, OSAP Prevention Monograph – 4. Rockville, MD: US Department of Health and Human Services.

Duffy M. (1987) Advertising and the inter-product distribution of demand. *European Economic Review* **31**, 1051–1070.

Duffy M. (1991) Advertising in demand systems: testing a Galbraithian Hypothesis. *Applied Economics* **23**, 485–496.

Farrell S. (1985) Review of National Policy Measures to Prevent Alcohol-Related problems. Geneva: World Health Organization (unpublished document PAD 85.14).

Franke G. and Wilcox G. (1987) Alcoholic beverage advertising and consumption in the United States, 1964–1984. *Journal of Advertising* **16**, 22–30.

Gerbner G., Gross L., and Morgan M. (1986) Living with television: the dynamics of the cultivation process. In: Bryant J. and Zillman D. (ed.) *Perspectives on Media Effects*, pp.17–40. Hillsdale, NJ: Laurence Erlbaum Associates.

Gerstein D. and Green L. (ed.) (1993) *Preventing Drug Abuse: What Do We Know?* Washington, DC: National Academy Press.

Giesbrecht N., Pranovi P., and Wood L. (1990) Impediments to changing local drinking practices: lessons from a prevention project. In: Giesbrecht N., Conley P., Denniston R. W., Gliksman L., Holder H., Pederson A., Room R., and

Shain M. (ed.) *Research, Action, and the Community: Experience in the Prevention of Alcohol and Other Drug* Problems, pp. 161–182, OSAP Prevention Monograph – 4. Rockville, MD: US Department of Health and Human Services.

Gliksman L. (1986) Alcohol management policies for municipal recreation departments: an evaluation of the Thunder Bay model. In: Giesbrecht N. and Cox A. (ed.) *Prevention and the Environment*, pp. 198–204. Toronto: Addiction Research Foundation.

Goodstadt M.S. (1978). Alcohol and drug education; models and outcomes. *Health Education Monograph* **6**, 263–279.

Goodstadt M.S. (1980) A turn on or a turn off? *Journal of Drug Education* **10**, 8–9.

Goodstadt M.S. (1989) Drug education: the prevention issues. *Journal of Drug Education* **19**, 197–208.

Goodstadt M.S. and Caleekal-John A. (1984) Alcohol education programs for university students: a review of their effectiveness. *International Journal of the Addictions* **19**, 721–741.

Grabowski H. (1976) The effects of advertising on the inter-industry distribution of demand. *Explorations in Economic Research* **3**, 21–75.

Grant M. and Room R. (1983) Potential media approaches to the prevention of alcohol-related problems. Paper presented at the Meeting of the World Health Organization, Geneva.

Graves K.S. (1992) Do warning labels on alcoholic beverages make a difference: a comparison of the United States and Ontario. *18th Annual Alcohol Epidemiology Symposium*, Toronto. 20 May–5 June.

Greenfield T.K., Graves K.L., and Kaskutas L.A. (1993) Alcohol Warning Labels for Prevention : National Survey Findings. *Alcohol, Health and Research World*, **17**, 67–75.

Grube J.W. and Wallack L. (1994) The effects of television beer advertising on children. *American Journal of Public Health*, **84**, 254–9.

Hankin J.R., Sloan J.J., Firestone I.J., Ager J.W., Sokol R.J., and Martier S.S. (1993) A time series analysis of the impact of the alcohol warning label on antenatal drinking. *Alcoholism: Clinical and Experimental Research* **17**, 284–289.

Hansen W.B., Johnson C.A., Flay B.R., Graham J.W., and Sobel J. (1988*a*) Affective and social influences approaches to the prevention of multiple substance abuse among seventh grade students: results from Project SMART. *Preventive Medicine* **17**, 135–154.

Hansen W.B., Graham, J.W., Wolkenstein B.H., Lundy B.Z., Pearson, J., Flay B.R., and Anderson J.C. (1988*b*) Differential impact of three alcohol prevention curricula on hypothesized mediating variables. *Journal of Drug Education* **18**, 143–153.

Hewitt L. E. and Blane H. T. (1984) Prevention through mass media communication. In: Miller P.M. and Nirenberg T.D. (ed.) *Prevention of Alcohol Abuse*, pp. 281–323. New York: Plenum Press.

Hilton M.E. (1992) Perspectives and prospects in warning label research, 18th Annual Alcohol Epidemiology Symposium, Toronto, 30 May – 5 June.

Hingson R., McGovern T., Heeren T., Winter M. and Zakocs R. (1993) Impact of the Saving Lives Program, 19th Annual Alcohol Epidemiology Symposium, Krakow, Poland, June.

Homel R. (1988) Random breath testing in *Australia: a complex deterrent. Australia Drug and Alcohol Review* **7** 231–241.

Iwaarden van M.K. (1983) Advertising, alcohol consumption and policy alternatives. In: Grant M., Plant M. and Williams A. (ed.) *Economics and Alcohol: Consumption and Controls*, pp. 223–237. London: Croom Helm.

Kohn P.M. and Smart R.G. (1984) The impact of television advertising on alcohol consumption: an experiment. *Journal of Studies on Alcohol* **45**, 295–301.

Kohn P.M. and Smart R.G. (1987) Wine, women, suspiciousness and advertising. *Journal of Studies on Alcohol* **48**, 161–166.

Kohn P.M., Smart R.G., and Ogborne A.C. (1984) Effects of two kinds of alcohol advertising on subsequent consumption. *Journal of Advertising* **13**, 34–48.

Lazarsfeld P.F. and Merton R.K. (1948) Mass communications, popular task and organised social action. In: Schramm W. (ed.) *Mass Communications*, pp. 492–512. Urbana, IL: University of Illinois Press.

Lee B. and Tremblay V. (1992) Advertising and the US market demand for beer. *Applied Economics* **24**, 69–76.

Lefler W. and Clark K. (1990) Drinksafe – a mass media alcohol education campaign. *Drug Education Journal of Australia* **4**, 165–177.

McCarty D. and Ewing J A. (1983) Alcohol consumption while viewing alcoholic beverage advertising. *International Journal of the Addictions* **18**, 1011–1018.

McCombs M.E. and Shaw D.L. (1972) The agenda-setting function of the mass media. *Public Opinion Quarterly* **36**, 176–187.

McGuiness T. (1980) An econometric analysis of total demand for alcoholic beverages in the UK. *Journal of Industrial Economics* **22**, 1215–27.

Mayer R.N. and Smith D.R. (1991) Utah Alcohol Warning Label Study: Consultants' Report to Medical Research Institute/Alcohol Research Group (unpublished manuscript, Salt Lake City, UT, University of Utah).

Mayer R.N., Smith K.R., and Scammon D.L. (1991) Evaluating the impact of alcohol warning labels. *Advances in Consumer Research* **18**, 1–9.

Mazis M.B., Morris L.A., and Swasy J.L. (1991) An evaluation of the alcohol warning label: Initial survey results. *Journal of Public Policy and Marketing* **10**, 229–241.

Milio N. (1986) Health and the media in Australia: an uneasy relationship. *Community Health Studies* **10**, 419–422.

Mills K.E., McCarty D., Ward J., Minuto L., and Patzynski J. (1983) A residence hall tavern as a collegiate alcohol abuse prevention activity. *Addictive Behaviour* **8**, 105–108.

Ministère des Affaires Sociales et de l'Integration (1991) *Dossier de Presse Prevention de l'alcoolisme. le 2 Decembre 1991*, p. 19.

Moskowitz J.M. (1989) The primary prevention of alcohol problems: a critical review of the research literature. *Journal of Studies on Alcohol* **50**, 54–88.

Muster E. (1985) Work with the media: the popular vote on drug advertising. In: Grant M. and Waahlberg, R. (ed.) *Extending Alcohol Education*, pp. 52–61. Lausanne: International Council on Alcohol and Addictions.

Ogborne A. and Smart R. (1980) Will restrictions on alcohol advertising reduce alcohol consumption? *British Journal of Addiction* **75**, 293–296.

Partanen J. and Montonen M. (1988) *Alcohol and the Mass Media*. EURO Reports and Studies 108. Copenhagen: World Health Organization. Regional Office for Europe.

Pentz M. A., Dwyer J.H., MacKinnon D.P., Flay B.R., Phil D., Hansen W.B., *et al.* (1989). A multicommunity trial for primary prevention of adolescent drug abuse. Effects on drug use prevalence. *Journal of the American Medical Association* **261**, 3259–3266.

Petty R. and Cacioppo J. (1981) *Attitudes and Persuasion: Classic and Contemporary Approaches*. Dubrique, IA: Wm. C. Brown.

Postman N., Nystrom C., Strate L., and Weingartner C. (1988) *Myths, Men, and Beer: an Analysis of Beer Commercials on Broadcast Television, 1987*. Falls Church: AAA Foundation for Traffic Safety.

Rogers E. M. and Shoemaker F.F. (1971) *Communication of Innovations*. New York: Macmillan.

Rubin A. (1986) Uses, gratifications, and media effects. In: Bryant J. and Zillman D. (ed.) *Perspectives on Media Effects*, pp. 1–16. Hillsdale, NJ: Erlbaum.

Saffer H. (1991) Alcohol advertising bans and alcohol abuse: An international perspective. *Journal of Health Economics* **10**, 65–79.

Saffer H. (1993) Alcohol advertising bans and alcohol abuse: reply. *Journal of Health Economics* **12**, 229–234.

Saffer H. (in press) Alcohol advertising and alcohol abuse: econometric evidence. *The Effects of the Mass Media on the Use and Abuse of Alcohol* (NIAAA Monograph).

Selvanathan E. (1989) Advertising and alcohol demand in the UK: further results. *International Journal of Advertising* **8**, 181–188.

Smart R.G. (1988) Does alcohol advertising affect overall consumption: a review of empirical studies. *Journal of Studies on Alcohol* **49**, 314–323.

Smart R.G. and Cutler R. (1976) The alcohol advertising ban in British Columbia: problems and effects on beverage consumption. *British Journal of Addiction* **71**, 13–21.

Sobell L.C., Sobell M.B., Riley D.M., Klajner F., Leo G.I., Pavan D., and Cancilla A. (1986) Effect of television programming and advertising on alcohol consumption in normal drinkers. *Journal of Studies on Alcohol* **47**, 333–339.

Staulcup H., Kenward K., and Frigo D. (1979) A review of federal primary alcoholism prevention projects. *Journal of Studies on Alcohol* **40**, 943–968.

Stewart L. and Casswell S. (1993) Media advocacy for alcohol policy support: results from the New Zealand community action project. *Health Promotion International* **8**, 167–175.

Strickland D.E. (1982) Alcohol advertising: orientations and influence. *International Journal of Advertising* **1**, 307–319.

Strickland D.E. (1983) Advertising exposure, alcohol consumption and misuse of alcohol. In: Grant J., Plant M., and Williams A. (ed.) *Economics and Alcohol: Consumption and Controls*, pp. 201–222. New York: Gardner Press Inc.

Taking Inititative: The 1990 Citizen's Movement To Raise California Alcohol Excise Taxes To Save Lives (1992) Washington DC: The Advocacy Institute.

Thorson E. (in press) Effects of alcohol advertising. *The Effects of the Mass Media on the Use and Abuse of Alcohol* (NIAAA Monograph).

Tobler N.S. (1986) Meta-analysis of 143 adolescent drug prevention programs: quantitative outcome results of program participants compared to a control or comparison group. *Journal of Drug Issues*, **16**, 537–67.

Wallack L.M. (1980) Assessing effects of mass media campaigns: an alternative perspective. *Alcohol, Health and Research World* **5**, 17–29.

Wallack L.M. and Barrows D.C. (1983) Evaluating primary prevention: the California 'winners' alcohol program. *International Quarterly of Community Health Education* **3**, 307–336.

Wallack L.M. (1990) Social marketing and media advocacy: two approaches to health promotion. *World Health Forum* **11**, 143–154.

Wilks J., Vardanega A.T., and Callan V.J. (1992) Effect of television advertising of alcohol on alcohol consumption and intentions to drive. *Drug and Alcohol Review* **11**, 15–21.

Worden J.K., Flynn B.S., Merrill D.G., Waller J.A., and Haugh L.D. (1989) Preventing alcohol-impaired driving through community self-regulation training. *American Journal of Public Health* **79**, 287–290.

Young O. (1993) Alcohol advertising bans and alcohol abuse: comment. *Journal of Health Economics* **12**, 215–228.

9

Individually directed interventions as a component of the public health response to alcohol

Twenty years ago scientists and practitioners concerned with treatment of drinking problems would generally have been viewed as standing at a distance from those working on the study and implementation of prevention. This distinction reflected differences in underlying assumptions as to what should count as 'the alcohol problem'. Treatment professionals probably saw the problem as 'alcoholism', but the prevention and public health experts were more likely to conceive the fundamental concerns as being at population level, in terms of the population's drinking behaviour and as embracing diverse and disaggregated alcohol problems. Within the contemporary thinking, there appeared to exist what Room (1977) was to call 'two worlds of alcohol problems'. Different views as to the central nature of the matter in hand were matched by contrasting theoretical discourse. Both at the level of national planning and community action, treatment and prevention were conceived, implemented, and assessed as largely unrelated activities.

This chapter will argue for a different and more holistic vision. A continuum of problems from minor to major, from single to multiple, from one-time events to sustained dependence or chronic illness, will require a continuum of responses. Within those responses treatment and prevention are complementary and often merged activities within the total public health activity. In Section 9.1 the logical basis for this position will be briefly analysed. Section 9.2 will examine research evidence for the efficacy of various types of treatment, in relation to their impact on the individual drinker. Evidence as to the possible summated benefits of individually directed interventions on the aggregate population will be discussed in Section 9.3. Finally, in Section 9.4, the overall direction of the policy implications of these diverse findings will be considered.

9.1 Individually directed interventions as a contribution to the overall public health approach to alcohol

9.1.1. *What interventions?*

For purposes of the present chapter we will use the phrase 'individually directed interventions' to embrace activities carried out by various agencies which have as a common feature the aim of intervening helpfully with the individual's drinking, or supporting those whose lives are affected by that drinking. The potential range of actors and actions involved is vast and disparate. As well as the activities of the primary care sector (Babor, *et al*. 1986), accident and emergency medicine, general hospitals (Chick, *et al*. 1985), psychiatric services, and specialist treatment units (Ettore 1984, 1985; Harris and Colliver 1989; Higuchi *et al*. 1991; de Silva *et al*. 1992), the list must, for instance, embrace the contribution made by social and welfare agencies; mutual help groups such as Danshukai in Japan, Kreuzbund in Germany, Croix d'or and Vie Libre in France, Abstainers Clubs in Poland; Links in Scandinavian countries, and AA and Al-Anon with their broad diffusion (Mäkelä 1991; Kurube 1992); workplace programmes (WHO 1993); court-mandated treatment for the drunk driver or other types of alcohol-related offence (see Chapter 7); the many efforts made by voluntary organizations to help the homeless drinker or the community at large (Argeriou and McCarthy 1990). For purposes of this review we will concentrate on those sectors where information on efficacy is more available, but that inevitably excludes much important background action. Assessment is needed not only of individual elements of intervention, but also of total, community-wide treatment systems, although research which addresses that level of analysis is still comparatively rare (Yahr 1988; Rush and Tyas 1990; Klingemann, *et al*. 1992). Between different countries patterns of care vary greatly, and thus the partition for instance between primary care and specialist treatment, between out-patient and in-patient care. Patterns which have been established in many developed countries with an emphasis on relatively costly specialist interventions are unlikely to be replicable in the developing world, but by far the greater part of the research literature again derives from the experience of industrialized countries. The research on primary care interventions which we will discuss later does, however, bridge developing and developed world feasibilities and experiences.

9.1.2 *Dissecting the multiple goals and impacts of interventions directed at individuals*

Individual intervention is always and primarily an act to help the individual, and that is its ethical and contractual basis. The relationship between prevention and treatment, and between individual level and public health perspectives is clarified, however, when the potentially multiple goals and impacts of the helping process are dissected thus:

1. *The impact of individually directed activity on public awareness and the setting of agenda.* The impact of a lay movement such as AA on public and political awareness has in the USA been important, despite the fact that AA rigorously avoids intentional political involvement. Less commonly remarked but also influential in many countries has been the willingness of the medical and related professions to become involved with these issues, and their consequent role as health advocates or community leaders (for instance, Royal College of Psychiatrists 1979). There are echoes here of matters discussed in Chapter 8 in relation to the wider societal impact of educational campaigns and community action – the possibility in the present instance is that mutual help organizations, the treatment professional, the 'recovered alcoholic' as neighbour, will very widely provide role models, educate the public, influence the media, impact on policy makers, or slowly change deeper societal awareness. There has, however, to date been little empirical research to assess these influences.

2. *Interventions with the goal of helping the individual drinker.* Here the aim may be, for instance, for the primary care professional to educate an individual patient on less risky drinking, or screen for risk factors which will be amenable to education. In such an instance, the health service worker is contributing directly to prevention, rather than acting in a conventional role and strictly as a provider of treatment. It is particularly this kind of extension to the previous range of health responses to drinking and drinking problems which breaks down the old demarcation between treatment and prevention. But the primary care practitioner or hospital doctor may, of course, also still be offering treatment to the individual in a conventional sense, with that treatment targeted at the drinking behaviour or the dependence, or at any one or more of many possible complications.

3. *Interventions directed at the drinking individual, but with the goal of protecting society or saving immediate societal costs.* All interventions which help the individual may be expected to offer indirect benefit to the family or the larger society. There are also though strategies which have as an intended component to these primary interventions, the achievement of second-order benefits. Drink driver (Wells-Parker *et al.* 1988, 1989) and workplace programmes (WHO 1993), and help directed at the pregnant

woman (Rosett *et al*. 1983; Larsson 1983; Schorling 1993), provide examples of this type of strategy.

4. *Interventions aimed directly at helping the person on whom the drinker's behaviour impacts*. Here some examples are provided by Al-Anon as a self-help group for family members or friends of individuals with drinking problems, and by recent lay movements concerned with the school-age children (Emshoff and Anyan 1991), or adult children of alcoholics (Brown 1991). The aim is to give direct help to the implicated person rather than the second-order type of effect discussed above.

So much for a brief analysis of the various types of impact which individually directed interventions may be intended to have on drinkers, on those immediately around them, and on society. Without abandoning the belief that treatment is an activity rooted in a responsibility toward the individual, this analysis inevitably points to the conclusion that individual interventions also in many ways have potential relevance to prevention, and to public policy, and for the larger public good.

9.2 Research evidence for the efficacy of individually directed interventions judged in terms of individual benefit

9.2.1 *Primary care and brief interventions*

Recent years have witnessed an extensive research output bearing on the issues defined by this heading, with reviews having been provided by Bien *et al*. (1993), Chick (1993), and Babor (in press). There is an overlap between the primary care and brief intervention research literature, but not all primary care intervention is 'brief', and brief intervention can be delivered other than in the primary care setting. For convenience, however, we will consider the two issues together.

Turning first to a study conducted within the primary care setting, Wallace *et al*. (1988) investigated 47 group practices in England to determine the effectiveness of advice given to heavy drinkers. Patients in the intervention condition received one session of advice to reduce their alcohol consumption, and the opportunity to participate in additional sessions. The intervention consisted of information feedback, specific advice to reduce alcohol consumption, a drinking diary, and a self-help booklet. The control group received no advice about drinking, except at their own request, or if there was evidence of significantly impaired liver function. Follow-up assessments at 6 and 12 months revealed significant reductions in both the control and the intervention groups, but there was a greater than twofold reduction in the intervention group compared with controls. These changes in reported alcohol consumption were corroborated by similar reductions in gamma-glutamyltransferase (GGT) levels, a liver enzyme test, in the male sample. The reduction in consumption was positively associated with the number of advice sessions attended.

Anderson and Scott (1992) conducted a randomized trial of brief interventions with male heavy drinkers identified at eight primary care group practices in the UK. Heavy drinkers and persons previously warned to cut down were excluded, qualifying this study as an early intervention trial. The intervention consisted of 10 minutes of advice about drinking, feedback concerning the results of a GGT test, and information about the risks of heavy drinking. A recommendation was made to consume no more than 24 grams of ethanol per day, or 168 grams per week. In comparison with an untreated control group, the intervention group at 1 year follow-up showed a small but statistically significant reduction in the quantity consumed and the proportion of heavy drinking days, as well as a 13% reduction in the proportion of heavy drinkers. A parallel study was conducted in a sample of women (Scott and Anderson 1990). At 12-month follow-up there was a significant reduction in the alcohol consumption of both the intervention and the control groups. The authors suggest that many women in the control group may have received advice from other sources to reduce their drinking.

A further example of brief intervention research comes from Sweden. Kristenson and his colleagues studied a group of middle-aged men who had been identified as 'heavy drinkers' as part of a general community-wide health screening project (Kristenson *et al.* 1982, 1983). Men identified as having an abnormal GGT reading were randomly assigned to either a counselling group or a control group. Although the GGT values of both groups decreased significantly, over a 6 year period the intervention group improved more in terms of absenteeism, sick days, and days hospitalized. Six years after the intervention there were small but significant differences in mortality. The study showed that simple intervention based on regular feedback about a biochemical marker had a beneficial effect on the drinking habits and physical health of a population considered at risk.

Still within the paradigm of brief intervention, in a major cross-national study sponsored by WHO (Babor and Grant 1992), a total of 1661 non-dependent heavy drinkers were recruited from a combination of hospital settings, primary care clinics, work sites, and educational institutions in cities in Australia, Bulgaria, Costa Rica, Kenya, Mexico, Norway, USSR, UK, USA, and Zimbabwe. Of these, 73% were evaluated approximately 9 months following random assignment to a control group, a simple advice group, or a group receiving brief counselling. The results showed a significant effect of the interventions on both average alcohol consumption and intensity of drinking in the male samples, even after controlling for demographic factors and socio-cultural influences. For females, significant reductions were observed in both the control and the intervention groups. The results also showed that the intensity of the intervention was not related to the amount of change in drinking behaviour, with 5 minutes of simple advice as effective as brief counselling.

The overall conclusion which emerges from this section of the review can be the robust assertion that brief interventions directed at excessive drinking, or at early stage alcohol problems, are likely to offer significant benefit to men. The situation as regards women is at present less clear, but it is difficult to believe that an absolute gender difference in responsiveness to advice of this kind is likely to exist.

There is also work which reports the application of rather more complex individually directed techniques with community samples, or the benefits from providing written self-help material to patients (Miller and Munoz 1976; Miller and Taylor 1980; Miller and Hester 1986), and there is additionally a positive report on the effectiveness of brief counselling in the general hospital setting (Chick *et al.* 1985).

9.2.2 *Evidence of individual benefit from specialized professional treatment of alcohol dependence*

The research issues raised by this heading are many and diverse, and we will not explore them in great detail. Recent reviews have been given by Miller and Hester (1986), Institute of Medicine (1990), and by Holder and Parker (1992). Views as to what constitutes appropriate treatment and hence the choice of outcome measures, will in part be culturally rooted (Babor 1986). The following general conclusions can be drawn from this complex body of evidence:

1. Subjects who have entered any kind of treatment will, 12 months later, probably show significant improvement over the pretreatment baseline, in relation to drinking and associated disabilities, but with considerable variations in outcome between samples. A direct causal effect of the treatment intervention cannot necessarily be imputed (Orford and Edwards 1977; Miller and Hester 1986).

2. Controlled trials give varied results, but there is no consistent evidence that intensive or in-patient treatment will give greater benefit than less intensive out-patient treatment (Orford and Edwards 1977; Miller and Hester 1986; Chick *et al.* 1988; Cook 1985*a,b*; Howden-Chapman and Huygens 1988; Postamianos *et al.* 1986; Drummond *et al.* 1990).

3. There is extensive literature on the relative efficacy of specific specialized treatments. Caution is needed against drawing any universal conclusions, given the heterogeneity of the treatment population, the many methodological problems involved, and the possibility that different factors may influence recovery in the shorter or longer term (Vaillant *et al.* 1985; Moos 1990; Edwards *et al.* 1992). The weight of evidence does, however, persuasively suggest that at least in the short- or medium-term, behavioural treatments are likely to be more effective than insight-oriented individual, group, or family therapies (Miller and Hester 1986; Saunders 1989).

4. The possibility of rational treatment/patient matching continues to attract interest, and there is some evidence to suggest that more intensive interventions may be more appropriate for the more dependent patient (Institute of Medicine 1990), although a recent report did not support this conclusion (Edwards and Taylor 1994).

5. The coexistence of various types of psychopathology may significantly influence the treatment needs and treatment responsiveness of the drinker (Meyer 1986), as may the presence of other drug problems (Galanter 1992).

In general, the available data on specialized treatment give some useful indications as to the likely overall merit of broadly different treatment approaches, but as already emphasized these results need to be interpreted within social context, and with awareness of the relatively brief time frame of most follow-up studies.

9.2.3 *Alcoholics Anonymous and evidence for its impact at individual level*

Although attempts have been made to assess the efficacy of AA through application of controlled design (Walsh *et al.* 1991), selection and other methodological difficulties pose problems for the interpretation of results. In many ways AA is both a 'treatment' and something very much more: a philosophy, a social movement, the offer of a friendship network, as well as a take-it-or-leave-it kind of walk-in treatment agency (McCrady and Miller 1993). It is therefore not too surprising that conventional research paradigms applied to assessment of its individual level efficacy have thus far not given meaningful results. Some might even argue that the essential nature of mutual help groups with their spontaneous, informal recruitment, defies randomization and controlled design, with compulsory assignment to AA not a test of AA as a self-help organization.

9.2.4 *Drinking driver rehabilitation programmes*

The use of education and rehabilitation as alternatives to court-imposed legal sanctions for people convicted of drinking–driving has increased steadily in many countries since the 1970s (Mäkelä *et al*. 1981). In some nations these programmes are used in lieu of traditional punitive sanctions such as jail, fines, or license revocation. In general, evaluation research conducted in the USA indicates at best a small effect of some interventions on recidivism and drinking behaviour (Wells-Parker *et al*. 1989). Given these modest effects, some have argued that the use of education and rehabilitation, while probably better than doing nothing at all, is not a suitable replacement for licencing sanctions (Hagen 1985). One study does, however, suggest that adding a rehabilitation programme to the sanctions has a beneficial effect (Mann *et al*. 1994).

9.3 Evidence for population level impact of individually directed interventions targeted at alcohol misuse

Here we return to the question of whether individual interventions can be shown to produce measurable population benefits through summation. Work which addresses this question is developing, but is still at a relatively early stage. In terms of extrapolation from the individual level findings, brief intervention in the primary care setting might be expected to provide a specially hopeful instance for follow-through to population effect, but at present there is only circumstantial evidence which bears specifically on that question (Holder *et al*. 1991). The available data relate to specialized treatment and to AA. Some reports deal with the population impact of these two interventions separately, while some take them together. Given the increasing numbers of problem drinkers involved in specialized treatment in the USA and in some other countries, it would indeed be reasonable to speculate that these programmes may have a significant impact on aggregate-level indicators of alcohol-related harm. For example, a recent survey of specialized treatment programmes in the USA (Weisner and Morgan 1992) identified approximately 6000 units, which were treating about 350 000 patients at the date of enquiry.

There is early evidence that treatment has the potential to produce aggregate impact. Several researchers have identified relationships between fall in liver cirrhosis rates and the growth of specialized treatment. Mann *et al*. (1988) found that decreased hospital discharges for liver cirrhosis were associated with increased treatment in Ontario, Canada, comparing 1975 and 1982 data. Romelsjö (1987) suggested that in addition to decreased per capita consumption, out-patient treatment may have accounted for the reduction in liver cirrhosis rates in Stockholm, Sweden. The evidence from both these studies is correlational and not particularly compelling in terms of the magnitude of the effects. However, a more recent study by Holder and Parker (1992) employed multivariate time-series analyses on the 20-year period 1968–1987 in North Carolina, and found a statistically significant reduction in cirrhosis mortality which could be attributed to increased alcohol treatment admissions (both in- and out-patient). These three studies from three different countries, provide promising support for aggregate level impact. The evidence of impact would be strengthened by replication in other countries.

If AA is effective in some cultures, then its impact on morbidity and mortality would depend on the number of members actively involved in its programmes. According to AA World Headquarters (1990), there were 46 400 groups in the USA in 1989. Membership is estimated to be approximately 1 million. In Canada, AA membership in 1983 was estimated to be 75% of the number of patients treated for alcohol problems in health care facilities (Smart, *et al*. 1989). To the extent that AA groups are more numerous than out-patient treatment, they may constitute a significant resource for drinkers who are attempting to reduce or stop drinking.

Researchers at the Addiction Research Foundation of Ontario (Smart *et al*. 1989; Smart and Mann 1990; Mann *et al*. 1991), found a relationship between AA membership and alcohol-related problems, including cirrhosis rates, in the USA, Canada, and other countries. Smart and Mann (1991) argued that in the USA and Canada the large reductions in liver cirrhosis rates are in part attributable to increased levels of AA membership. Smart and Mann (1990) concluded that increased treatment and AA membership could have accounted for a substantial proportion of the reductions in cirrhosis deaths and hospital discharges in Ontario and in the USA between 1975 and 1982. Mann *et al*. (1991) estimated that a 1% increase in AA membership would be associated with a 0.06% decrease in cirrhosis mortality. They concluded that 'large increases in AA membership would be necessary to justify an expectation of substantially reduced cirrhosis deaths'. These three North American studies do not establish causality but provide correlational evidence to suggest the potential of AA membership to affect cirrhosis at an aggregate level. If, however, these relationships are in some degree causal, the implication is that with greater availability of treatment and AA, alcoholic cirrhosis could be reduced significantly.

There have been a series of studies in the USA which provide evidence that treatment of people with drinking problems produces a reduction of total health care costs. These findings which span some 20 years in a variety of treatment populations, support the cost–benefit potential of such interventions (Longabaugh *et al.* 1983; Holder 1987; Holder and Blose 1992; Holder *et al.* 1992).

In summary, research on the population impact of individually directed interventions does not as yet give conclusive answers, but these questions are only beginning to be addressed.

9.4 Pointers for policy: treatment and prevention as seamless response

At the beginning of this chapter reference was made to the degree of disjunction between the prevention and treatment policy worlds which existed 20 years ago. On the basis of the research which has been reviewed above, the argument that this type of segmentation in many ways fails to meet present realities and needs, would seem to be amply supported. A perception of the problems as a continuum, proposes by a logical symmetry a continuum of policy responses, to which prevention and treatment contribute in overlapping and mutually supportive fashion. Health care is founded in commitment to helping the individual, but manifestly the health care agent or agency may usefully contribute to interventions directed at risky drinking which constitute a type of prevention pure and simple, and primary prevention within the conventional definition. At the same time interventions offered to the individual will, of course, constitute secondary or tertiary prevention. We have also discussed the immediate benefits for those individuals affected by the drinker, and the likelihood that treatment activity may enhance the level of public awareness on alcohol problems. The existence of treatment services and the witness borne by the recovered drinker may importantly contribute to public awareness and willingness to support other policy action. Treatment must never lose its roots in commitment to helping the person, but research begins to hint that help to the individual may show through at the level of related population morbidity and mortality, and presumably therefore also in terms of social costs.

For treatment to achieve significant population benefit it must be widely available within the population, and its costs, complexity, and acceptability must be such as to make dissemination feasible. Services will need to respond both to acute and long-term problems. More intensive and expensive treatment does not necessarily mean better results; low-cost alternatives can assist substantially with early identification, secondary prevention, and long-term support. Those alternatives are epitomized by the primary care interventions and mutual help organizations discussed in this chapter.

References

Alcoholics Anonymous World Headquarters (1990) *1989 Membership Survey*. New York: AA World Services.

Anderson P. and Scott E. (1992) Randomized controlled trial of general practitioner intervention in men with excessive alcohol consumption. *British Journal of Addiction* **87**, 891–900.

Argeriou M. and McCarthy D. (1990) *Treating Alcoholism and Drug Abuse among Homeless Men and Women: Nine Community Demonstration Grants*. New York: Haworth.

Babor T.F. (ed.) (1986) *Alcohol and Culture: Comparative Perspectives from Europe and America*. Annals of the New York Academy of Sciences, Vol. 472. New York: The New York Academy of Sciences.

Babor T.F. (1994) Avoiding the horrid and beastly sin of drunkenness: does dissuasion make a difference? *Journal of Consulting and Clinical Psychology* (in press).

Babor T.F. and Grant M. (1992) *Project on Identification and Management of Alcohol-related Problems. Report on Phase II: A randomized clinical trial of brief interventions in primary health care*. Geneva: World Health Organization.

Babor T.F., Ritson, E.B., and Hodgson R.J. (1986) Alcohol-related problems in the primary health care setting: a review of early intervention strategies. *British Journal of Addiction* **81**, 23–46.

Bien T.H., William R., and Tonigan S. (1993) Brief interventions for alcohol problems: a review. *Addiction* **88**, 315–336.

Brown S. (1991) Adult children of alcoholics: the history of a social movement and its impact on clinical theory and practice. In: Galanter M. (ed.) *Recent Developments in Alcoholism*, Vol. 9. *Children of Alcoholics*, pp. 267–286. New York: Plenum.

Chick J. (1993) Brief interventions for alcohol misuse. *British Medical Journal* **307**, 1374.

Chick J., Lloyd G., and Crombie E. (1985) Counselling problem drinkers in medical wards: a controlled study. *British Medical Journal* **290**, 965–967.

Chick J., Ritson R., Conaughton J., Stewart A., and Chick J. (1988) Extended treatment for alcoholics: a controlled study. *British Journal of Addiction* **83**, 625–634.

Cook C.C.H. (1985a) The Minnesota Model in the management of drug and alcohol dependence: miracle, method or myth? I. The philosophy of the programme. *British Journal of Addiction* **80**, 625–634.

Cook C.C.H. (1985b) The Minnesota Model in the management of drug and alcohol dependence: miracle, method or myth? II. Evidence and conclusions. *British Journal of Addiction* **80**, 735–748.

Drummond D.C., Thom B., Brown C., Edwards G., and Mullan M.J. (1990) Specialist versus general practitioner treatment of problem drinkers. *Lancet* **336**, 915–918.

Edwards G. and Taylor C. (1994) A test of the matching hypothesis: alcohol dependence, intensity of treatment, and 12 month outcome. *Addiction* **89**, 553–61.

Edwards G., Oppenheimer E., and Taylor C. (1992) Hearing the noise in the system: exploration of textual analysis as a method for studying change in drinking behaviour. *British Journal of Addiction* **87**, 73–81.

Emshoff J.G. and Anyan L.L. (1991) From prevention to treatment: issues for school-aged children of alcoholics. In: Galanter M. (ed.) *Recent Developments in Alcoholism*, Vol. 9, *Children of Alcoholics*, pp. 327–346. New York: Plenum.

Ettore E.M. (1984) A study of alcoholism units – 1. Treatment activities and the institutional response. *Alcohol and Alcoholism* **19**, 243–255.

Ettore E.M. (1985) A study of alcoholism treatment units: some findings on links with community agencies. *British Journal of Addiction* **80**, 181–189.

Galanter M. (1992) *Recent Developments in Alcoholism*, Vol. 10. *Alcohol and Cocaine. Similarities and Differences*. New York: Plenum.

Hagen R.E. (1985) Evaluation of the effectiveness of educational and reha-bilitation efforts. Opportunities for research. *Journal of Studies on Alcohol* Suppl.10, 179–183.

Harris J.R. and Colliver J.D. (1989) Highlights from the 1987 National Drug and Alcoholism Treatment Unit Survey (NDATUS). *Alcohol Health and Research World* **13**, 178–182.

Higuchi S., Muramatsu T., Yamada K., Muraoka H., Kno H., and Eboshida A. (1991) Special treatment facilities for alcoholics in Japan. *Journal of Studies on Alcohol* **52**, 547–554.

Holder H. (1987) Alcoholism treatment and patient health care cost saving. *Medical Care* **25**, 52–70.

Holder H. and Blose J. (1992) The reduction of health care costs associated with alcoholism treatment: a 14-year longitudinal study. *Journal of Studies on Alcohol* **53**, 293–302.

Holder H. and Parker R.N. (1992) Effect of alcoholism treatment on cirrhosis mortality: a 20-year multivariate time series analysis. *British Journal of Addiction* **87**, 1263–1274.

Holder H., Longabaugh T., Miller W.R., and Rubonis A.V. (1991) The cost effectiveness of treatment for alcoholism. A first approximation. *Journal of Studies on Alcohol* **52**, 517–540.

Holder H., Lennox R., and Blose J. (1992) The economic benefits of alcoholism treatment: a summary of twenty years of research. *Journal of Employee Assistance Research* **1**, 63–82.

Howden-Chapman P.C. and Huygens I. (1988) An evaluation of three treatment programmes for alcoholism: an experimental study with 6- and 12-month follow-up. *British Journal of Addiction* **83**, 67–81.

Institute of Medicine (1990) *Broadening the Base of Treatment for Alcohol Problems*. Washington, DC: National Academy Press.

Klingemann H., Takala J-P., and Hunt G. (1992) *Cure, Care or Control: Alcoholism Treatment in Sixteen Countries*. Albany, NY: State University of New York Press.

Kristenson H., Ohlin H., Hulten-Nosslin M., Trell E., and Hood B. (1983) Identification and intervention of heavy drinkers in middle-aged men: results and follow-up of 24–60 months of long-term study with randomized controls. *Alcoholism: Clinical and Experimental Research* **7**, 203–209.

Kristenson H., Trell E., and Hood B. (1982) Serum of glutamyl-transferse in screening and continuous control of heavy drinking in middle-aged men. *American Journal of Epidemiology* **114**, 862–872.

Kurube N. (1992) National models: self-help groups for alcohol problems not applying the Twelve Step program. *Contemporary Drug Problems* Winter, 689–715.

Larsson G. (1983) Prevention of fetal alcohol effects: an antenatal program for early detection of pregnancies at risk. *Acta Obstetricia et Gynecologica Scandinavica* **62**, 171–178.

Longabaugh R., McCrady B., Fink E., Stout R., McAuley T., Doyle C., and McNeill D. (1983) Cost effectiveness of alcoholism treatment in partial vs. inpatient settings: six month outcomes. *Journal of Studies on Alcohol* **44**, 1049–1071.

McCrady B.S. and Miller W.R. (ed.) (1993) *Research on Alcoholics Anonymous: Opportunities and Alternatives*. New Brunswick, NJ: Alcohol Research Documentation, Inc. Rutgens Center for Alcohol Studies.

Mäkelä K. (1991) Social and cultural preconditions of Alcoholics Anonymous (AA) and factors associated with the strength of AA. *British Journal of Addiction* **86**, 1405–1413.

Mäkelä K., Room R., Single R., Sulkunen, P., and Walsh B. (1981) *Alcohol, Society and the State*, Vol. 1. Toronto: Addiction Research Foundation.

Mann R.E., Smart R., Anglin L., and Rush B. (1988) Are decreases in liver cirrhosis rates a result on increased treatment for alcoholism. *British Journal of Addiction* **83**, 683–688.

Mann R.E., Smart R., Anglin L., and Adlaf E. (1991) Reductions in cirrhosis deaths in the United States: associations with per capita consumption and AA membership. *Journal of Studies on Alcohol* **52**, 361–365.

Mann R.E., Anglin L., Wilkins K., Vingilis E.R., Macdonald S., and Sheu W-J. (1994) Rehabilitation for convicted drinking drivers (second offenders). Effects on mortality. *Journal of Studies on Alcohol*, forthcoming.

Meyer R.E. (ed.) (1986) *Psychopathology and Addictive Disorders*. New York: Guildford.

Miller W.R. and Hester R.K. (1986) Matching problem drinkers with optimal treatments. In Miller W.R. and Heather N. (ed.) *Treating Addictive Behaviors: Processes of Change*, pp. 175–203. New York: Plenum.

Miller W.R. and Munoz R.F. (1976) *How to Control Your Drinking*. Englewood, NJ: Prentice-Hall.

Miller W.R. and Taylor C.A. (1980) Relative effectiveness of bioliotherapy, individual and group self-control training in the treatment of problem drinkers. *Addictive Behaviours* **5**, 13–24.

Moos R.H., Finney J.W., and Cronkite E. (1990) *Alcoholism Treatment: Context, Process and Outcome*. New York: Oxford University Press.

Orford J. and Edwards G. (1977) *Alcoholism. A comparison of Treatment and Advice, with a Study of the Influence of Marriage*. Maudsley Monograph, No.26. Oxford University Press.

Postamianos G., North W.R.S., Meade T.W., Townsend J., and Peters T.J. (1986) Randomised trial of community-based centre versus conventional hospital management in treatment of alcoholism. *Lancet* **ii**, 797–799.

Romelsjö A. (1987) Decline in alcohol-related in-patient care and mortality in Stockholm County. *British Journal of Addiction* **82**, 653–663.

Room R. (1977) Measurement and distribution of drinking patterns and problems in general populations. In: Edwards G., Gross M.M., Keller M., Moser J., and Room, R. (ed.) *Alcohol-Related Disabilities*, pp. 61–88 WHO Offset Publication No. 32. Geneva: WHO.

Rosett H.L., Weiner L., and Edelin K.C. (1983) Treatment experience with pregnant problem drinkers. *Journal of the American Medical Association* **249**, 2029–2033.

Royal College of Psychiatrists (1979) *Alcohol and Alcoholism*. London: Tavistock.

Rush B.R. and Tyas S.L. (1990) *Alcohol and Other Drug Services in Ontario: Results of a Provincial Survey, 1989*. Toronto: Addiction Research Foundation.

Saunders J. (1989) The efficacy of treatment for drinking problems. *International Review of Psychiatry* **1**, 121–138.

Schorling J.B. (1993) The prevention of prenatal alcohol use: a critical analysis of intervention studies. *Journal of Studies on Alcohol* **54**, 261–267.

Scott E. and Anderson P. (1990) Randomized controlled trial of general practitioner intervention in women with excessive alcohol consumption. *Australian Drug and Alcohol Review* **10**, 311–322.

Silva de H.J., Peiris, M.U.P.K., Samarasinghe D.S., and Ellawala N.S. (1992) A two-year follow-up study of alcohol dependent men rehabilitated at a special unit in a developing country. *British Journal of Addiction* **87**, 1409–1414.

Smart R. and Mann R.E. (1991) Factors in recent reductions in liver cirrhosis deaths. *Journal of Studies on Alcohol* **53**, 232–240.

Smart R. and Mann R.E. (1990) Are increases in treatment levels and Alcoholics Anonymous membership large enough to reduce liver cirrhosis rates. *British Journal of Addiction* **85**, 1291–1298.

Smart R., Mann R.E., and Anglin L. (1989) Decreases in alcohol problems and increased Alcoholics Anonymous membership. *British Journal of Addiction* **84**, 507–513.

Vaillant G.E. (1983) *The Natural History of Alcoholism*. Cambridge, MA: Harvard University Press.

Wallace P., Cutler S., and Haines A. (1988) Randomised controlled trial of general practitioner intervention in patients with excessive alcohol consumption. *British Medical Journal* **297**, 663–668.

Walsh D.C., Hingson R.W., Merrigan D.M., Levenson S.M., Cupples L.A., Heeren T. *et al.* (1991) A randomized trial of treatment options for alcohol-abusing workers. *New England Journal of Medicine* **325**, 775–782.

Weisner C. and Morgan P. (1992) Rapid growth and bifurcation: Public and private alcohol treatment in the United States. In: Klingemann H., Takala J.P., and Hunt G. (ed.) *Cure, Care or Control: Alcoholism Treatment in Sixteen Countries* pp. 223–252 Albany, NY: State University of New York Press.

Wells-Parker E., Anderson B.J., Landrum J.W., and Snow R.W. (1988) Long-term effectiveness of probation, short-term intervention and LAI administration for reducing DUI recidivism. *British Journal of Addiction* **83**, 415–421.

Wells-Parker E., Anderson, B.J., McMillen D.L., and Landrum J.W. (1989)

Interactions among DUI offender characteristics and traditional intervention modalities: a long-term recidivism follow-up. *British Journal of Addiction* **84**, 381–390.

WHO (1993) *Health Promotion in the Workplace: Alcohol and Drug Abuse.* Report of an Expert Committee. Geneva: WHO.

Yahr H.T. (1988) A national comparison of public and private-sector alcoholism treatment delivery system characteristics. *Journal of Studies on Alcohol* **49**, 233–239.

10

The policy implications

Without trivializing the complexities or forcing answers where uncertainty exists, the task now is to identify how the evidence presented earlier in this book can be brought sharply into focus on policy options. There are findings which can usefully and generally illuminate, as opposed to dictate, policy decisions in diverse settings. Alcohol policies should be based on the best possible interpretation of these findings rather than on misinformation, muddle, and rhetoric. Beyond any doubt the evidence in sum demonstrates factually and forcefully that measures are available which can significantly reduce the burden of alcohol-related harm.

This chapter will be structured in the following way. Section 10.1 will recapitulate a set of conclusions, which provide the background for an understanding of alcohol as a policy issue. Section 10.2 explores how research can practically inform the front line of policy choice. Section 10.3 looks briefly at how a policy mix is best to be achieved and prioritized. Section 10.4 is short. It tries to meet that always difficult challenge, 'Write down on a couple of sheets of paper the core of your conclusions.'

We intend this chapter as a summary mapping of the issues which we would like to put before policy makers. It will not be referenced, but reference back will be made as appropriate to section numbering in previous chapters.

10.1 Alcohol as a public health issue: the basis of understanding

10.1.1 *The target problems are pervasive and enormously costly*

On a world scale drinking results in diverse suffering and costs of enormous proportion which have an impact on the health and welfare of men and women; children and adults; the poor and the rich; those who do the drinking and those who suffer from the drinker's behaviour, in nearly every country of the globe. Alcohol is a highly significant public health issue, but with intersecting significance for health services, welfare, family protection, youth, employment and productivity, public order, road safety and crime, agriculture, trade, and revenue and taxation (Sections 1.3 and 1.4).

Any belief that alcohol is a circumscribed problem because, supposedly, its 'misuse' only affects a small minority of the population who can be tidied away and classified as deviants or 'alcohol abusers', is mistaken. Those countries which at present have low problem rates would do well to protect their relative advantage rather than taking present comfort as basis for unguardedness.

10.1.2 *Neither a country's level of drinking nor its experience of drinking problems are immutable*

That the level of a population's alcohol problem experience is not set for all time is a fact of crucial significance to policy formation, providing as it does both warning and reason for optimism. Data presented in Section 1.4.1 demonstrate enormous geographical differences in cirrhosis death rate, while at other points in this book evidence has been presented to show that both drinking behaviour, and drinking problems, vary over time (Chapter 2). In many countries, what happens in this arena is for the most part not shaped by intentional health and social policy, but by drift or economic determinant alone.

The message for the policy process to be drawn from this evidence, is that it will in every sense be expensive to leave the level of a country's experience with alcohol problems to chance. Drinking and drinking problems will in part be influenced over time and for better or worse, by background cultural and social influences which are not susceptible to public health action. The tide is though to a significant extent controllable, and to give substance to this contention is, of course, the thrust of this book and the matter for summary in 10.2.

10.1.3 *Quantity drunk and problems experienced in a given population are generally related*

Chapter 3 has presented evidence at the individual level which establishes a dose–response relationship between alcohol intake and malignancies (Section 3.6.1), blood pressure and stroke (Section 3.6.2), cardiac conditions (Section 3.6.3), and liver cirrhosis (Section 3.6.4). There is a relationship between individual alcohol consumption and road traffic accidents (Section 3.7), and individual consumption is associated with other types of accidents, violence towards others, suicide, and likelihood of being a victim of attack (Sections 3.7 and 3.8). Volume, and frequency of the individual's heavy drinking, are related to adverse social consequences (Section 3.8). Individual consumption is related to likelihood of a person experiencing alcohol dependence (Section 3.9). Overall mortality risk shows a J-shaped relationship with consumption (Section 3.10), but beyond a modest level of intake, more drinking implies a heightened overall mortality risk. *The individual's level of drinking is thus significantly related to the risk of that individual encountering a problem with alcohol.*

The analysis of the relationship between the individual's drinking and individual risk given in Chapter 3, is followed in Chapter 4 by material which establishes the relationship between the population's level of drinking and the population problem experience. A basis is established for understanding population problem occurrence through the interaction between individual risk and distribution of consumption levels within the population (Section 4.1). Population consumption is shown to be related to aggregate mortality among middle-aged men to the extent that a 1 litre increase in per capita consumption will be reflected in a 1% increase in mortality (Section 4.3.2). There is a significant relationship between population consumption level and population mortality from cirrhosis, alcoholic psychosis, alcoholism, pancreatitis, and certain cancers (Sections 4.3.3 and 4.3.4). There is mixed evidence on the relationship between population consumption and traffic fatalities (Sections 4.3.5). There is a positive relationship between overall consumption and suicide, and between consumption and violence toward others (Section 4.3.6). *The overall level of a population's drinking is significantly related to the level of alcohol-related problems which that population will experience.*

Thus in sum and standing back from the detail, a strong and multiple linkage exists between drinking and drinking problems. That assertion is today supported by overwhelming research evidence and when policy decisions are being made, sight should not be lost of this finding. Policies should be shaped within an awareness that except for a reduced risk of coronary heart disease mortality at low levels of intake, more drinking by the individual is likely to put that person at greater risk of incurring an alcohol-related problem, while more drinking by a population will carry an added burden of aggregate alcohol-related damage.

These assertions do not derive from any natural law, but from consistencies in the findings of empirical research. From these consistencies there are likely to be some exceptions which will helpfully assist understanding of the processes which shape the consumption and problems relationship. Thus pattern as well as quantity of drinking may often have to be taken into account (Section 3.3.1). The setting in which the drinking takes place may bear on individual risk (Section 3.8). Age may interact with drinking to determine driving risk (Section 3.7). Drinking is not a behaviour which exists in isolation, but one which may interact with other life-style behaviours such as smoking, diet, and exercise (Section 3.3.3). Culture influences drunken comportment, with consequent population-level variations in the relationship between alcohol and, for instance, suicide (Section 4.3.6). It is theoretically possible to envisage intentional strategies which would alter the relationship between mean consumption and population distribution of drinking, but this is in practical terms likely to be difficult to achieve. In the long-term it is also possible that drinking norms will change within a given population in response to background social influences, with shifts in patterns of population drinking distribution. *Generally, however, increase in per capita consumption will be followed by an increase in drinking across the drinking population, and an increase in the number of heavy drinkers (Section 4.2), with consequences for rate of any particular problem depending on the curvature of the risk function (Section 4.3).*

10.1.4 *The problems which alcohol policy targets should be broadly defined*

The policy target should not be limited to 'alcoholism', the alcohol addict, or extreme physical illness. The target definition which will best inform policy development will take cognizance both of alcohol-related problems and alcohol dependence; it will give high priority to acute and accident problems as well as chronic pathologies; it will deal with social and psychological, as well as physical problems (Section 1.3). It will deal with small and common problems as well as major and less common consequences. Policy must be concerned with the adverse impact of the drinking on the family and other people as well as on the drinker. Drink-driving (Chapter 7) and other aspects of alcohol-related crime, come within the target definition.

Research furthermore demonstrates that policy must be willing to take the totality of the drinking population as defining the scope for public health action. *Society's drinking problems will on the large scale be dealt with effectively through understanding and influencing the total and dynamic system which comprises society's drinking, and effective policies cannot be modelled exclusively in terms of picking off little pieces of the continuum, or trying to manipulate extremes of behaviour.* The evidence which underpins this assertion is of two kinds, and can be summarized thus:-

1. *Prevention measures which influence the generality of drinkers will often also impact on heavy or problematic drinkers (Sections 4.2.3, 4.2.4, 4.3., 6.3.1)* The drinking population in general behaves as one system rather than as several different parts. Increase or decrease in overall consumption is therefore likely to result in shifts across all bands of drinking, and will have an impact on heavy drinkers who are already experiencing problems, or who are especially vulnerable to risk of encountering problems.

2. *Many of the target problems are widely distributed in the drinking population, rather than being concentrated only among heavy drinkers.*

Policies targeted at the larger sector of a population manifesting lesser degrees of individual risk, but in sum containing many problems, can for some problems produce greater public health benefit than a focus on a smaller population at higher risk but with in sum a lower yield of problems. This is referred to as the 'Prevention Paradox', but this argument does not apply to all types of alcohol-related problem, and again it is necessary to take into consideration the shape of the risk curve (Section 4.1.1).

10.2 The research evidence and the levers of policy

This section will bring together evidence on how the research which has been reviewed in previous chapters, and the principles which have been summarized above, can inform practically the choice of policy option. The purpose is not to be prescriptive, but, echoing the intentions stated at the beginning of the book, to offer guidance as to how research can empower the policy process. Our intention here is to help identify the potential policy levers and give some indication as to which are likely to be most powerful.

10.2.1 *The aim of alcohol policies which are implemented within this arena must be to reduce the occurrence of problems*

To support that broad aim two interactive and mutually supportive types of policy will be required. First it will be necessary to operate measures which bear on consumption. What is being proposed here is a means to an end and should not be construed as an end in itself. The overall strategy must create an environment which helps people to make healthy choices and renders unhealthy choices more difficult or expensive. *But if the level of alcohol consumption is allowed to run free and go high, more targeted interventions will be rendered null and void.* The second type of policy response is concerned with responses targeted at specific high risk contexts or behaviours.

Any measures which will potentially increase the availability of alcohol within a country, whether as a result of trade agreements, reduction in real price of beverage alcohol, or reduction or elimination of restrictions on retail access, should therefore be judged in terms of public health and public safety, in addition to any other perspectives. This observation is of particular importance to currently less industrialized countries where social and economic developments can easily lead to a large and steep upsurge in alcohol availability. This same general point is also relevant to countries where former government restrictions on retail sales controls through the operation of state monopolies or licensing systems, are tending to be relaxed. That having been said, the perspective which is being developed here stresses the need for balance: alcohol availability and aggregate-level responses cannot be the sole focus, more targeted measures are not by themselves a sufficient policy response, but when put intelligently together these two kinds of approach will jointly and synergistically support the aim of reducing alcohol problems. We return to the question of policy mix in Section 10.3.

10.2.2 *Taxation of alcohol is an effective environmental mechanism for reducing alcohol problems broadly*

There is abundant evidence that the population's alcohol consumption is responsive to price (Chapter 5). Through the relationship between consumption on the one hand and individual and population problems on the other (Chapters 3 and 4), taxation of alcohol is a public health lever of wide potential effectiveness. To argue that heavy or dependent drinkers will be immune to the influence of price is to argue against the facts. Furthermore, the reasoning set out above in 10.4 provides the basis for taking the broad drinking population as the target for problem prevention. *Put simply, but with entire scientific accuracy, alcohol taxation is an effective and readily available environmental policy instrument which can be applied to save lives and avert alcohol-related suffering.* Any country which intends to take the prevention of alcohol problems seriously must ensure that in determining the level of taxation, health interests are represented and taken into account.

10.2.3 *Environmental measures which influence physical access to alcohol can make a significant contribution to prevention of alcohol problems*

Such measures include enactment of a minimum legal drinking age; restrictions on hours or days of sale; and policies on number, type, or location of sales outlets. These and similar measures should not be viewed in isolation, but as elements in a coherent alcohol control policy which structures the alcohol market so as to limit consumption. In some countries, these measures have traditionally been the province of a specific alcohol control agency. *Research demonstrates the effectiveness of these kinds of environmentally directed measures, but they should again be viewed as a means to a policy end, rather than as restrictiveness for restriction's sake.* By the same token, these useful contributions to the total public health response should not be dismantled piecemeal because political sentiment turns against restrictiveness, with the reasons for such measures having been introduced in the first place forgotten (Chapter 6).

10.2.4 *Drink-driving countermeasures are effective if vigorously enforced and given a high public profile*

Drink-driving provides an encouraging instance of the rational, stepwise application of scientific findings to policy development (Chapter 7). This topic also illustrates the vital importance of policy intentions being backed by a sustained commitment to making them work. *Drink-driving counter-measures will not achieve results through token intention, but when enforced and publicly seen to be enforced, they can prevent accidents and save lives.* Overall consumption will bear on drink-driving, and hence taxation and access measures are again here relevant.

There are a number of approaches which may make it less likely that people will drink and drive. Deterrence and the strict enforcement of drink-driving laws (7.1) is of fundamental importance. Other measures include server training, making the person or premises which supply the drink to an intoxicated patron legally liable (Sections 6.3.9 and 6.3.10), or schemes whereby a nominated person in a social group agrees not to drink (Section 7.2). Mandated treatment or AA referral of the convicted driver do not appear to have much impact on recidivism (Section 7.1.4).

10.2.5 *Other situationally directed measures*

Policy experience is developing in relation to other situationally directed prevention measures – control of alcohol sales at football matches, for instance (Section 7.5).

10.2.6 *School-based education, public education, warning labels, and advertising restrictions*

These policy elements have in common the intention of influencing the individual's knowledge, attitudes, and behaviour (Chapter 8). They are interventions which are by their nature likely to be interactive with many other environmental influences, and if they have an impact it is likely to be in the longer term (Section 8.1). Their longer-term efficacy is difficult to research, but if they have benefit, it is perhaps more likely to be indirect and through heightened political and public awareness (Section 8.2). *There is no present research evidence which can support their deployment as lead policy choices or justify expenditure of major resources on school-based education or mass media public education campaigns*, unless these are placed in a broader context of community action.

10.2.7 *Indicative personal drinking limits as a health education strategy*

Thus far there is no evidence to support the efficacy of campaigns which as a public health strategy seek to teach the population to count the number of units of alcohol which they drink (Section 8.1.2). Furthermore, there may be some danger that talking about a 'safe limit' will encourage wider population drinking and spur light drinkers to drink up to the stated limit. In both developing and developed countries, the majority of the population are likely to be drinking below any promulgated 'safe limit'. The evidence discussed in Chapter 3 shows that for several adverse consequences, no safe limit but a continuity of risk exists. The point has though also been made that risk does not increase until a level of about three standard drinks a day for either men or women is reached, but because of the possible risk for cancer of the female breast any limit for women should be set lower, at say two drinks a day. Various further objections to the limits concept can be entered: failure to take individual body weight and other aspects of individual vulnerability into the reckoning; failure to emphasize the importance of style, pattern, and spacing of drinking; failure to deal with the importance of drinking context. Furthermore, in Section 4.1.3, the highly important policy point is made that the optimum health limit for population drinking is, because of variance around the mean, considerably lower than any putative individual level.

All in all, it would seem best to talk about 'lower risk limits' than 'safe limits' (Section 3.10). Although the concept is useful for discussion between doctor and patient and for setting and monitoring of individual drinking goals, as the basis for campaigns which seek to set or influence population drinking behaviour, the approach is not likely to be helpful.

10.2.8 *The association between light drinking and reduced risk of coronary heart disease*

Evidence on the protective effect of drinking on coronary heart disease is conclusive at the level of association, highly suggestive at the level of causation, but not on present analysis significant at the policy level (Sections 3.5.1 and 4.1.3). Most of the achievable benefit is likely to be obtained at an alcohol intake between one drink every 2 days, and two drinks a day. There are other public health measures for prevention of coronary disease of far more persuasive effectiveness than encouragement of drinking. *Any attempt to put about a message which encourages drinking on the basis of hoped-for gains in coronary heart disease prevention, would be likely to result in more harm to the population than benefit.*

10.2.9 *Community action programmes*

A variety of community action programmes have been reported (Section 8.1.3). These have often been multifaceted and provided a context for both environmentally directed interventions and information giving strategies. This is a relatively new research area. The evidence to date is not extensive but suggests some potential for comprehensive community action to reduce alcohol problems. However, it seems likely that *the community's acceptance of, or better still its active backing, is a prerequisite for the successful application of any public health policy*, and must be integral to alcohol policies. Community action strategies recognize this fact, and aim to mobilize existing community resources and support to this end.

10.2.10 *The contribution which treatment can make to public health policies*

In designing policies to deal with drinking problems, to split off prevention and treatment as separate spheres of activity is unhelpful. *Treatment can tangibly support public health goals in this arena* (Chapter 9). It is often difficult to obtain public interest and support for other public health policies if the need for adequate treatment is ignored. If alcohol treatment is to make a significant, population-wide impact on drinking problems it must though be delivered on an appropriate and community-wide scale. Different levels and types of problem may require different types and degrees of intervention, and policies cannot be based on the assumption that there is any one treatment which is appropriate for every drinking problem. Strong evidence points though to the frequent effectiveness of simple help given in general or primary care settings (Section 9.2.1), and the importance of the primary care response to drinking and drinking problems deserves strong emphasis.

10.3 Making the policy mix and defining policy priorities

We have in 10.2 summarized evidence on a variety of policies which have as their common goal a reduction in the burden of alcohol problems. In each instance we have tried to give an indication of the likely degree of efficacy. To go further and attempt to determine how policies should be optimally mixed or prioritized in any particular country, raises questions which can only properly be answered by authorities within the individual country setting. We offer below some notes to assist the policy maker who is facing this kind of responsibility.

1. There is no one policy panacea. *Alcohol problems have multiple causes, arise in many different situations, and affect diversities of people. Inevitably, therefore, the needed policies will be a mix rather than a master-stroke.*

2. In general, the research strongly points to some policy measures as being more likely to produce the wanted effect than others. A policy mix which makes use of taxation and control of physical access, which supports drink-driving countermeasures, and which invests broadly in treatment and particularly in primary care, is on all the research evidence likely to achieve success in reducing the level of problems. Educational strategies or restrictions on advertising can be added to that mix, but that must be on the basis of reasonable hope of long-term pay-off, rather than evidence of the kind which supports the former group of strategies. There is early evidence that public education campaigns can increase awareness, and thus public support for other environmental policies. Comprehensive community action programmes may also have potential. To design a policy mix which gave salience to education directed at individual drinking while neglecting strategies of proven worth would, however, run counter to the research conclusions and cannot be expected to succeed.

3. Political feasibility and public acceptance are of inevitable importance in selecting alcohol policies. Feasibility and acceptance are not, however, fixed quantities. The evidence for the scope, seriousness, and costs of the target problems has to be stated, and the public educated better to understand the logical case for policy choice. Drink-driving again provides a telling case in point. Public education on the nature of the policy issues is part of the policy job.

4. Policy choices will today often need to take cognizance of an international dimension. Achieving a health input to international trade or tariff agreements and dealing with the alcohol trade across borders may often today be highly important if the best national alcohol policy intentions are not to be negated.

5. Policy choices will as ever have to be determined not only by what is effective, but what gives value for money. There is as yet little information on the relative cost-effectiveness of different alcohol policies, and we have not discussed that question in this book. The issue will though need to be addressed when making choices.

Although there is now wide and widely researched policy experience on which to build, every choice or mix of policy is a new experiment.

Continued monitoring and assessment of interventions in this arena must be a prudent part of the total effort.

10.4 Summing it all up

One reply to the challenge to 'write it on a couple of pages' would be to duck the invitation and mandate everyone else to compose their own statement – a truly participatory exercise. We will, however, briefly attempt to say what in essence we see as the distillate of the message which we hope the intended audience will take away from this book.

1. Alcohol problems have too often been left to ebb and flow. It is the job of policy so far as possible to capture and control that tide in the public interest.

2. We believe that the title of this book is well chosen. Policy to deal with the multifarious consequences stemming from alcohol cannot usefully be couched in terms just of 'excessive drinking' or 'right-hand end of the curve' policies disarticulated from the whole society, nor in terms just of 'alcohol problem policies', or 'How are we to deal with alcoholics?'. The requisite public policies are, in the round, alcohol policies.

3. Behind the statistics there lies much suffering and heavy cost. The plea that alcohol issues should be given higher policy priority is manifestly justified.

4. Alcohol gives pleasure as well as pain, and any government which fails to acknowledge that fact is unlikely to take the people with it.

5. The quality and astonishing scope and international spread of the research output which has been presented in this book indicates that public health policies on alcohol have today a strong evidential underpinning. We argue and recommend from a basis of considerable factual weight which derives from a sustained scientific endeavour. The research establishes beyond doubt that public health measures of proven effectiveness are available to serve the public good and support the intentions of any administration that is determined to curb the widespread costs and pain which can be related to the use of alcohol. Science in this arena provides knowledge which can and should be used to the public good.

6. The fundamental aim of policy is to reduce alcohol problems, and all measures employed should be a means to that end. To that end, it will be appropriate to deploy responses both of a kind which influence

consumption and aggregate-level problems, and policies which are targeted on specific contexts and behaviours. To conceive of these intrinsically complementry approaches as contradictory alternatives would be unhelpful and mistaken.

7. Not all policies are likely to be equally effective, and on the basis of the research evidence discriminating policy choices should be made. In this arena not all measures are equally good, and to put heavy investment into relatively ineffective policies is wasteful and diversionary.

8. The tone within which alcohol issues are discussed is important. We would plead that there is now sufficient science in this arena for policies to be rationally rooted. Doctrinaire passion and vested interest are equally poor guides to decision making where so much is at stake, and where ample research is now available to inform the policy process.

9. There should be acknowledgement of the continuing gaps in knowledge. If research is better to empower the policy process, there is still many a research mile to go.

Those of us who have worked together in collegiate fashion on the preparation of this book will feel well rewarded if its impact is to stimulate very broadly a strengthened commitment and sense of rational optimism in relation to problems which have too often in the past been viewed as intractable, been responded to only half-heartedly, or been left to the flow of the tide. Drinking problems are not carried by an uncontrollable tide. With public will, and on the evidence, they are capable of amelioration.

Appendix: research opportunities

In this appendix we will first outline the case for strengthening the geographic coverage of alcohol research. Secondly, a list will be given of what we perceive as being the leading further research opportunities. The aim is not to provide a comprehensive prospectus, but to give a view on where broad future strategic opportunities may lie.

1. The need to strengthen the international coverage of alcohol research

In this book rather little research has been cited which emanates from developing countries, from eastern Europe, or from the republics of the former USSR. Given the problems which may confront the establishment of a health research base in certain national situations, it is unsurprising that alcohol studies should not so far have secured more of a presence. Despite these difficulties and the problems of disseminating research findings, interesting individual pieces of work have appeared and deserve acknowledgement.

As was argued in Chapter 1, many policy relevant research findings are likely to generalize across countries, but at the same time countries which are in a state of rapid social, economic, and political change, are often encountering special problems with alcohol which interact with those happenings. Against that background there are two types of reason for believing that alcohol research deserves increased investment. There are first internal considerations relevant to these countries themselves, and alcohol policies in these settings as anywhere else need to be underpinned by research. There are then also reasons which are external: research which reflects the experience with alcohol in these parts of the world will contribute usefully, and at times vitally, to the sum of international understanding.

To make such a research policy recommendation is easier than identifying the funding and trained personnel to support the proposed investigations. Without entering into the specifics of an organizational solution, we would suggest that international agencies should be willing to assist in the establishment and support of the needed alcohol research capacity as an integral part of health planning. This need should also be drawn to the attention of national agencies in countries which offer training assistance to the developing world.

2. Some emerging opportunities for policy-relevant alcohol research

These opportunities can be seen as lying within three domains which are to an extent overlapping.

2.1 *Studies of alcohol policies*

2.1.1 *The genesis of alcohol policies.* Such research can be expected to assist understanding of policy feasibilities or barriers to effective policy formation, in national or regional situations. We need to know more about how policies are actually made, and how to enable more effective public health policy on alcohol to develop in the real world.

2.1.2 *The design of models to predict the public health impact of different alcohol policies.* Work is needed on the design of models which can provide policy makers with projections as to the likely quantitative impact of particular public health measures, alone or in combination, on stated parameters of alcohol-related harm.

2.1.3 *Tariffs and trade agreements.* As mentioned in Chapter 5, tariff and trade agreements affecting the price and supply of alcohol are likely to be of increasing global importance. The impact of such developments on drinking and public health are therefore significant research issues.

2.1.4 *Treatment systems as a public health component.* Using the term 'treatment' as broadly employed in Chapter 9, there is a need for further work on the aggregate-level impact of such interventions, specially in relation to the population-level effect of penetration and diffusion of primary care.

2.1.5 *Cost-effectiveness of different alcohol policy choices.* Too little is at present known about either the cost, or cost-effectiveness, of different prevention or treatment options deployed in the alcohol arena.

2.1.6 *Studies of liquor industry policies.* The operation of national and multinational liquor industries is a legitimate research issue for health. Topics are likely to include the economics of production, and of beverage diversification; advertising, marketing and distribution, and the increasing internationalization of markets; association of the industry with other types of product (e.g. tobacco); lobbying and public relations strategies.

2.2 Studies on the nature of drinking behaviour and determinants of change in such behaviour

2.2.1 Definition and measurement of dimensions, or typologies, in patterns of drinking behaviour.   Further investment is needed in the conceptualization and measurement of *patterns* of alcohol use, and of transitions between patterns.

2.2.2 The interaction of multiple factors in determining change over time in individual drinking behaviour.   A great many research issues are subsumed under this heading. To break new ground the needed approaches will be likely to include research which explores the interaction between macro-level economic changes affecting aggregate population drinking, microsocial influences, and personal status including personal income, baseline individual drinking, and degree of alcohol dependence.

2.2.3 Closer understanding of the behaviour of different sectors within an overall drinking population.   We need to know more about what sectors of the population, in changing circumstances, drink less or more. The plea here is that we get beyond an overall population behaviour (a focus which has been scientifically profitable), and give more attention to changes in behaviour among subgroups defined by, say, gender, age, ethnicity, urbanization, income, baseline drinking, and alcohol dependence. The intention would be to establish a better understanding of the interactive dynamics of the 'drinking collectivity'.

2.3 Alcohol and alcohol-related problems

2.3.1 Accidents, casualty occurrences, interpersonal violence, and suicide.   There are an array of issues under this heading which have in common the fact that they are acute adverse consequences. The relationship between these problems and personal and aggregate-level drinking and drinking patterns, together with the interaction of setting, cultural and social influences, and personal characteristics, needs to be further understood.

2.3.2 Alcohol and chronic physical illness.   More needs to be known about the impact of drinking patterns, duration of alcohol exposure, congeners, dilution or type of beverage, modifiers such as dietary factors or smoking, and risk curves for the types of physical illness considered in Chapters 3 and 4. Cancer of the female breast in particular requires further attention of this kind.

2.3.3 *Public health implications of alcohol dependence.* Dependence has until recently been seen as largely a clinical concept rather than one applied in analysis of population-level issues. Research is now needed to explore the potential significance of this construct to the understanding of population drinking. Clarification is required as to the relationship between population drinking level and population prevalence of dependence. It will also be important to determine whether once established, a cohort of dependent drinkers will have a certain degree of entropy in their behaviour, thus influencing aggregate population behaviour.

2.3.4 *Alcohol and social problems.* Evidence has been presented that risk function analysis is possible for certain social problems both in relation to individual and aggregate drinking (Chapters 3 and 4). We suspect that further research in this area will in particular be strengthened by measurement of pattern as well as quantity of drinking, with other interactive influences taken into account.

2.3.5 *Alcohol and protection against heart disease.* Work is required on the levels and patterns of drinking which may impact on coronary disease, and the lower threshold and 'window' for any beneficial impact. Methodological issues relating to the measurement of long-term alcohol exposure require further attention. Further definition is needed of population subgroups which are more or less likely to benefit from a protective effect, and on the interaction with cigarette smoking.

3. Research options and the broad, continuing international alcohol research effort

Finally, we would wish again to emphasize that this listing of opportunities is not intended as exhaustive. There is a vital need for better, and more complete and integrated collection of data on issues such as alcohol consumption and alcohol-related mortalities and morbidities, and on social and legal problems. These data should be made widely available to researchers and policy makers, nationally and internationally. Research and health planning in relation to alcohol need not, and should not, be impeded by lack of reliable information. There is much need for continuation in existing lines of research such as, for instance, work directed at the policy topics identified in Chapters 5–9, and case studies in policy experience and the description of experiments of nature will go on being of great importance. Research methods and statistical techniques must be further developed in many areas. More than anything, research in this practical, theoretical, multidisciplinary area, has to be an open enterprise, with ability to respond to new and unexpected research opportunities as they arise.

Index